KU-266-823

PREVENTING
CANCERS

Edited by
Tom Heller, Lorna Bailey
and Stephen Pattison
at The Open University

CARLISLE

HAROLD BRIDGES LIBRARY
S. MARTIN'S COLLEGE
LANCASTER

Open University Press in association with the Open University

This Reader forms part of the Open University course P578 *Reducing the Risk of Cancers*. For further information on the course, write to the Department of Health and Social Welfare (P578), The Open University, Walton Hall, Milton Keynes MK7 6AA

This Reader is one part of an Open University integrated teaching system and the selection is therefore related to other material available to students. It is designed to evoke the critical understanding of students. Opinions expressed in it are not necessarily those of the course team or of the University.

Academic Editors: Tom Heller, Lorna Bailey, Stephen Pattison

Course Manager: Simon Baines

Course Secretary: Tanya Hames

Editors: Jill Alger, Kathy Eason

Designer: Siân Lewis

Graphic Artist: Roy Lawrance

EDUCATION CENTRE LIBRARY

CUMBERLAND INFIRMARY

CARLISLE CA2 7HY

512316

Open University Press
Celtic Court
22 Ballmoor
Buckingham MK18 1XW
England

and
1900 Frost Road, Suite 101
Bristol, PA 19007, USA

First published in 1992

Selection and editorial material copyright © 1992 The Open University

All rights reserved. No part of this publication may be reproduced, stored in a retrieval system or transmitted, in any form or by any means, without written permission from the publisher or a licence from the Copyright Licensing Agency Ltd. Details of such licences (for reprographic reproduction) may be obtained from the Copyright Licensing Agency Ltd, 90 Tottenham Court Road, London W1P 9HE.

Edited, designed and typeset by The Open University

Printed and bound in the United Kingdom

A catalogue record of this book is available from the British Library

Library of Congress Cataloguing-in-Publication number available

ISBN 0-335-19003-0 (pbk)
ISBN 0-335-19004-9 (hbk)

CONTENTS

LIST OF CONTRIBUTORS

Joan Austoker	Cancer Research Campaign, Oxford University, UK
Philippe Autier	Institut Jules Bordet, Belgium
Marc Buyse	International Institute for Drug Development, Belgium
Margo Dijkstra	University of Limburg, Holland
Julie Evans	Cancer Research Campaign, Oxford University, UK
Steven Greer	The Royal Marsden Hospital, UK
Angela Hall	London Hospital Medical College, UK
E. Heseltine	International Agency for Research on Cancer, France
Michael Henderson	Michael Henderson Research, Australia
Michael Hill	ECP (UK), UK
Donald C. Iverson	AMC Cancer Research Centre, USA
Martin J. Jarvis	Institute of Psychiatry, UK
Manolis Kogevinas	International Agency for Research on Cancer, France
Gerjo Kok	University of Limburg, Holland
Elsebeth Lynge	Danish Cancer Registry, Denmark
Rona M. MacKie	University of Glasgow, UK
Klim McPherson	London School of Hygiene & Tropical Medicine, UK
Roger Milne	*New Scientist*, UK
Calum Muir	Information & Statistics Division, Scottish Health Service, UK
Pascal Piedbois	Hôpital Henri Mondor, France
Allyson Pollock	Newham Health Authority, UK
James O. Prochaska	University of Rhode Island, USA
E. Riboli	International Agency for Research on Cancer, France
L. Shuker	International Agency for Research on Cancer, France
Malcolm Taylor	University of Birmingham Medical School, UK
Harri Vainio	Institute of Occupational Health, Finland
Hein de Vries	University of Limburg, Holland
Verner Wheelock	Verner Wheelock Associates Limited, UK
Patti White	UK
J. Wilbourn	International Agency for Research on Cancer, France

ACKNOWLEDGMENTS

Grateful acknowledgment is made to the following sources for permission to reproduce material in this reader.

Cover taken from Jaroff, L. 'Stop that Germ' in *Time*, May 23 1988;

2.3 Vainio, H. 'Occupational Cancer Prevention' in *Journal of Cancer Research and Clinical Oncology*, no. 113, 1987;

2.7 Heseltine, E., Riboli, E., Shuker, L. and Wilbourn, J. *Tobacco or Health: Warning: tobacco causes cancer and other fatal diseases – Smoke Free Europe* series no. 4, World Health Organisation for Europe, 1988;

3.3 Prochaska, J. O. 'What Causes People to Change from Unhealthy to Health–Enhancing Behaviour?' in *Cancer Prevention Journal*, Vol. 1, no. 1, pp. 38–42, © by Williams and Wilkins, 1990;

4.1 Iverson, Prof. D. C. 'Program Principles Associated with Successful Health Promotion Interventions' in *Human Behaviour and Cancer Risk Reduction*, August 1989.

INTRODUCTION

Despite all the intense research activity internationally in the therapeutic and clinical arenas over the last century, it now seems unlikely that a single definitive cure for cancers will ever be discovered. Knowledge and understanding about cancers is slowly and surely advancing. Pushing at the limits of therapeutic knowledge provides small increments of advantage and better chances of longer survival for the treatment of people who have one of the cancers, but it will probably never provide a speedy or conclusive solution for these diseases.

In the same way increasing knowledge about the causes of cancers is developing slowly and surely, making prevention more possible. The search for the causes of cancers and ways of preventing them depends on painstaking and complex multi-professional investigation. Through the efforts of workers in many disciplines throughout the world, mechanisms and factors in causation are being identified. It is thus becoming possible to use this increased understanding to intervene more effectively in practice in order to prevent cancers occurring and to reduce the risk of cancers for individuals and whole populations.

The aim of this book (and of the Open University (UK) course, P578 *Reducing the Risk of Cancers* of which it is a part) is to help health professionals and policy-makers throughout Europe and beyond to understand many of the elements of effective cancer prevention. With this increased knowledge and understanding they will be equipped to change the ways they work and be more effective in their activities designed to prevent more cancers from occurring in the future.

Internationally, there is an enormous amount of research and preventive activity, hence the international authorship of this volume. The papers that have been drawn together here represent many of the areas in which research

and analysis is helping to expand understanding of the preventability of cancers.

Although there are still many areas of ignorance and dispute in cancer causation and prevention, it is clear that much is already known which can form a reasonably solid base for action. While it is impossible to provide dogmatic answers to all questions about causation and effective prevention, the cumulative picture emerging from these papers is one of increasing optimism and encouragement for primary prevention. It is important to respond to the challenge of this activity now, for inaction in the present will ensure continuing and unnecessarily high rates of cancer incidence into the future. Enough is known about many of the major cancers to be able to advocate practical prevention strategies that will make an impact on future incidence and mortality.

Action to prevent cancers is most effectively situated within a framework of health promotion. Activity is required at many different levels to reduce the incidence of cancers; it is not just individuals who have to change their ways. A previous collection of papers about cancer prevention (Heller *et al.*, 1989) detailed the ways that governments, companies and communities have all got a part to play in the work to reduce the incidence of cancers. This belief underpins the present volume.

Another important assumption made throughout this volume is that individuals and social groups must be helped to improve their knowledge about risk management if change to more healthy ways of behaving is to be achieved. Better risk management based on sound knowledge, rather than paternalistic coercion, is seen as the key to effective and appropriate health promotion. Individuals must have the knowledge, freedom and resources to examine their own behaviour.

Where action is required at other levels, a full understanding of the current state of biomedical and epidemiological knowledge is important for policy- and decision-makers if they are to act responsibly and to bring about change in a progressive direction.

Engaging with the subject of cancer prevention is a stimulating and exciting challenge. Health care professionals and health policy decision-makers who have daily evidence of the problems and suffering that many types of cancers still cause are in the forefront of activities to reduce the burden of many cancers throughout Europe. The papers in this volume have been commissioned from a wide range of experts to equip health professionals in the field to develop their health promotion activities.

The nature and structure of this book

This book has been compiled from papers which help to build up a picture of the current state of knowledge about the causation of cancers and the actions required to prevent them. Most of the papers have been specially commissioned for this collection from a range of acknowledged experts in this field. A few of them have previously been published in medical journals, conference proceedings or elsewhere.

The authors, drawn from five European countries as well as from the USA and Australia, are all authorities on their various subjects. They present the latest overview of their topics. At all points, the implications of knowledge and research for preventive action are drawn out, making this volume a practical aid to cancer prevention.

Many of the papers describe examples of good practice in cancer prevention. Where doubt and uncertainty remain in a particular area, authors have been asked to clarify issues and to discuss problems in such a way that readers

will be able to understand them and join in the current debates about the best way forward.

The book is divided into four main parts. The papers in the first two parts focus on the ways in which international data from a variety of disciplines can build up a picture of the patterns of common cancers and the potential for preventing cancers. The first part, Finding Out What Causes Cancers, examines what is known about the causes of common cancers and details the epidemiological, sociological and biomedical factors which bear upon this. The second part, Preventable Cancers: Some Case Studies, deepens this approach by examining the causal factors bearing upon particular kinds of cancers and the implications of these findings for effective preventive interventions.

The challenge for all health care professionals posed by research into the causes of cancers is to find ways of working with individuals and with whole communities which actively change patterns of cancer incidence and bring about a reduction in mortality and morbidity from these cancers. The papers in the final two parts of the book start to address this issue. Helping Individuals Manage their Risk of Cancers is the theme of the third part. Here the focus is on how individuals can be helped to manage their risks of cancers, and questions such as 'What sort of interventions are appropriate?' and 'How do we know what will help and be effective?' are considered. The final part of the book, Integrated Action to Prevent Cancers, deals with other types of action to prevent cancers. Issues of policy, health promotion intervention and integrated action are examined in this part.

References

Heller, T., Davey, B. and Bailey, L. (eds.) (1989) *Reducing the risk of cancers*, Hodder & Stoughton, London.

PART 1

FINDING OUT WHAT CAUSES CANCERS

INTRODUCTION

The papers in this part of the book focus on basic epidemiological, sociological and biological understandings which are relevant to determining what causes cancers.

Social patterns of cancer distribution

The papers by Manolis Kogevinas and Elsebeth Lynge discuss the social patterns of cancer distribution, and search within these patterns for clues about the causation of particular cancers and how they might be prevented.

In 'Social inequalities and cancers', Kogevinas describes and discusses the social inequalities which can be demonstrated in cancer distribution. Especially amongst men, there is a pronounced inverse relation between the incidence of many cancers and social class position. This pattern of unequal distribution of cancers is present amongst unemployed men also. It is related to, but appears greater than, that explained by the patterns of known risk behaviour, such as tobacco and alcohol consumption, dietary intake and occupation itself. These findings pose the questions 'In what ways precisely do social variables bear on cancer causation?' and 'Why do lower class people enjoy poorer health over such a wide range of conditions including many cancers?' Kogevinas suggests that research into social inequalities in cancer distribution is useful for public health action, for research strategy (it helps to clarify factors of causation) and for theory insofar as it helps to relate social organization and structure to measurable levels of health and illness.

Kogevinas' perceptions are complemented by those of Lynge from the Danish Cancer Registry, one of the most effective and comprehensive cancer registries in the world. Drawing upon Danish and British data, in 'The importance of the social dimensions of cancer', Lynge describes factors such as age, social class and occupation as key variables in cancer causation. She points out that the social history of a country can have a large effect on the patterns of cancers that develop. She describes how overall rates of some cancers amongst men in Denmark have increased since they have gradually moved away from agricultural work, and makes the observation that the social class gradient in cancer causation is not uniform; Danish building workers have higher rates of lung cancer than farm workers who technically are classified as being in the same social class. Finally, Lynge raises issues about social evolution: 'If the entire Danish population had the same cancer risk as farmers, one-third of the cancer cases in males, and one-quarter of the cancer cases in women would not occur'. This is intriguing, because the way of farm life which is the background for these previously low cancer figures is now disappearing. Lynge highlights the fact that the change of social structure over time will have an effect on types and numbers of cancers in the future. Where the rates of some cancers are greater in men of higher social class, for example bowel cancer amongst academics compared with manual workers, this might give clues about the perils associated with sedentary lifestyles.

Finding out what causes cancers involves both descriptive and analytical epidemiology, looking at the patterns of cancer distribution and attempting to determine what causes them. It can also involve experimental research, making particular interventions to try to see if any introduced changes can affect these patterns. Marc Buyse *et al.* in their paper

'Clinical trials in cancer prevention' survey the methodological problems which arise in trying to find out whether specific interventions are successful in changing the patterns of cancer. Clinical trials are becoming increasingly important in the attempt to establish the causes of many cancers. They are also used to test out various interventions to see if they are effective in reducing the burden of mortality and morbidity from specific cancers. The paper outlines some of the difficulties in constructing scientifically valid studies of intervention because of factors such as the length of time such studies would take, the cost of undertaking them, the number of people who would have to take part in them, the dangers of contamination and other changes amongst subjects taking part. Despite these inherent problems, many clinical trials of cancer prevention are under way throughout Europe and they continue to add to the existing knowledge of the causes of cancers and what can be done to prevent them from occurring.

The work of building up comprehensive pictures of cancer epidemiology depends on good data. Calum Muir's paper 'Reliability of cancer data' assesses the types and reliability of cancer-related information which are available. Accurate knowledge of the incidence, prevalence and mortality rates associated with various cancers is vital in understanding the causes of cancers and when monitoring different types of preventive activity. Muir points to the difficulties associated with acquiring various types of accurate cancer data. In the case of mortality data, for example, there are problems of patchy coverage within populations, inadequate recording of deaths, and different coding systems used by different countries which makes international comparison problematic. The user of mortality data should therefore always ask the question 'Are death registration data complete and are they accurate?' In the case of incidence data, there are similar problems: data are sparse and there are often difficulties with under-reporting. In some countries, cancer registries cover all the population, but in others there is only partial coverage. This poses problems for getting to know more about the specific causes of cancers and should add to the pressure for the establishment of comprehensive cancer registries as a priority throughout Europe.

Biological aspects

In 'A simplified biology of cancers', Malcolm Taylor reviews current knowledge of the genetic basis of cancers which has emerged from extensive recent research. While the volume of research into the biological factors in carcinogenesis has been costly and intense, it is only slowly developing into an increased understanding of some of the mechanisms involved in cancer formation. This paper summarizes current knowledge about genetic and biological triggers for cancers and will help health professionals increase their own knowledge of the events leading to the formation of a cancer. This is important in helping them in their task of explaining these factors to people who seek their help and advice.

SOCIAL INEQUALITIES AND CANCERS

Manolis Kogevinas

Differences in cancer occurrence in England and Wales

Men in the lower social classes have a clearly higher incidence of all neoplasms than those of higher socio-economic status. An extensive investigation of differences in cancer incidence applying five different measures of socio-economic status (housing tenure, house amenities, car ownership, education and social class) showed that this pattern is apparent irrespective of the socio-economic classification used (Fox and Goldblatt, 1982; Moser *et al.*, 1986; Kogevinas, 1990). Cancer incidence by social class (Figure 1) indicates a steady increase in incidence of all neoplasms from social class I (professional) to social class V (unskilled manual workers); the latter have

an approximately 40% higher risk than the former. This variability by social class is apparent in nearly all age groups.

In women, differences in cancer are not as pronounced as in men, and women in the manual social classes have only a slightly higher incidence of all neoplasms than those in the non-manual social classes. Age standardized incidence ratios by social class based on women's own occupation are shown in Figure 2. A similar pattern is seen when restricting analysis to married women and classifying them by their own, or their husband's, occupation or when applying other socio-economic classifications. This overall picture shows, however, considerable diversity when examining social inequalities for specific cancers.

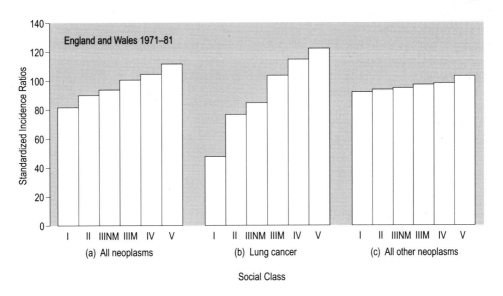

Figure 1 Social class differences in incidence of all neoplasms, lung cancer, and all other neoplasms except lung, among men

Women are classified by own social class and those in non-manual occupations are taken as the reference group

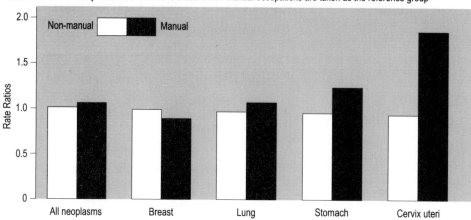

Figure 2   Social class differences in incidence of major cancers among women.
England and Wales 1971–81

A summary of socio-economic differences in men and women for specific cancers is shown in Table 1. It has been abstracted from an IARC publication (IARC, 1990a) and is based on an international comparison of social inequalities in cancer (Logan, 1982). In most countries and at most periods in time, men of lower socio-economic status have been found to have a higher incidence of, or mortality from, oral cancers, cancer of the oesophagus, stomach, liver, larynx and lung, while men in the higher social classes have higher incidence of malignant melanoma, cancer of the testis, brain, and Hodgkin's disease. Bladder cancer incidence has frequently been found to be higher in the lower social classes while the opposite pattern has been observed for colon cancer and the leukaemias; evidence for these three sites has not been consistent over time.

In England and Wales, the widest socio-economic differences with regard to the most common cancers in males are currently observed for cancer of the stomach and the lung. Differences in lung cancer incidence by social class for England and Wales, are shown in Figure 1(b). The increase in incidence by social class is very steep and men in social class V have two and a half times the risk of

men in social class I. Lung cancer accounts for approximately 30% of all male cancers, and it therefore contributes a large part of the socio-economic differences observed in cancer overall. This is clearly illustrated in Figure 1(c) which shows social class variation in all other cancers, except lung. An increasing gradient from social class I to social class V can still be observed, but the slope of the increase is very much attenuated. Social class differences for stomach cancer are even steeper than lung cancer; unskilled manual workers have about six times higher incidence than professionals.

Women of low socio-economic status have consistently been found to have higher incidence for cancer of the oesophagus, stomach, larynx, lung and cervix uteri, while for oral cancers and cancer of the liver there is little information available (Table 1). Women in the higher social classes have higher incidence of breast and ovarian cancer, and an incidence of malignant melanoma, Hodgkin's disease, brain tumours and the leukaemias similar to men. In women the widest differences with regard to the most common cancers are observed for cancers of the cervix uteri and of the stomach (Figure 2).

Table 1 Socio-economic differentials for selected cancer sites based on cancer mortality in the UK*

Site	Sex	Differential type	Variation over time	Further details
Buccal cavity and pharynx	M	Negative, moderate	Narrowing of differentials	Salivary gland is only component of site aggregate to show a negative differential in most studies.
	F	? Negative	No systematic change	Few available data
Oesophagus	M	Negative, moderate	Negative gradient has become steeper and smoother	
Stomach	M	Negative, strong	Constant despite sharp decline in mortality rate	One of the strongest and most consistent relationships with socio-economic position
	F			
Colon	M	? Positive	Positive gradient apparent to and including 1951; subsequently no relationship with social class seen	Strong positive differentials observed in studies of colon cancer in Cali, Colombia, and in Hong Kong; no consistent relationship seen in other recent studies
	F			
Rectum		No evidence of consistent differential		
Liver	M	Negative, weak	In early period, non-linear relationship seen; negative gradient most apparent in 1971	Few available data
	F	? Negative	No systematic change	Few available data
Pancreas		No evidence of consistent differential		
Larynx	M	Negative, strong	Relatively constant negative gradient maintained	Negative differentials seen in earliest available data, in contrast to lung cancer
	F			

Site	Sex	Differential type	Variation over time	Further details
Lung	M	Negative, strong	Social class differentials first apparent in 1951 for males and 1961 for females; gradient steepest in 1971	Outside of England and Wales, negative differentials seen for males and females in 1940s. In general, some evidence that male differentials wider than female differentials
	F			
Malignant melanoma	M	Positive, moderate	Differential slightly wider for females in 1971 than in 1961 or 1951. No earlier data available	Few available data
Breast	F	Positive, weak	Sharp narrowing of differential 1931–61. Small positive differential remaining for married and single women in 1971	Small positive differentials found with great consistency
Cervix	F	Negative, strong	Slight widening of differentials for married and single women 1951–71; no earlier data available in disaggregated form	Earliest socio-economic differential observed; almost always the largest differential reported in any study; found with complete consistency in every population investigated
Other uterus (principally corpus uteri)	F	No evidence of consistent differential		
Ovary	F	Positive, weak	Narrowing of differentials 1931–61; small positive differential remaining for married and single women in 1971	Similar pattern to breast, particularly with narrowing of differential over time; positive differential found in most studies
Prostate	M	Variable	Pronounced positive gradient in 1911 diminished with time to produce suggestion of weak negative gradient in 1971	Results of different studies contradictory

Site	Sex	Differential type	Variation over time	Further details
Testis	M	Positive, strong	Large positive differential remained relatively constant 1921–71	Positive differential shows consistency; however, few data available from decennial supplements
Bladder	M	Variable	Basic negative differential developed into smooth negative gradient between 1921 and 1971	Negative differential seen in decennial supplements is not confirmed in other studies, some of which indicate the existence of a positive differential, while others show no relationship with socio-economic position
	F			
Brain	M	Positive, weak	Early pronounced positive differential narrowed over time, leaving a small but perceptible positive differential in 1971	Positive differential found in most studies
Leukaemia	M	? Positive	Weak positive differential seen in most periods	Results of different studies are inconsistent; decennial supplements indicate that differentials may vary according to type of leukaemia
	F			
Hodgkin's disease	M	Positive, weak	Clear positive gradient in 1951 absent or only weakly present later	Some confirmation of positive differential from US data

*Positive differential: mortality higher in high social class.
Negative 433333 differential: mortality lower in high social class.

Source: Adapted from Logan (1982).

Social inequalities in cancer in other countries

Social class differences in cancer incidence in countries of northern and western Europe reveal a similar pattern to that seen in England and Wales; lung, stomach and cervical cancer are among those sites where wide differences are observed (Desplanques, 1976; Lynge, 1979; Vagero and Persson, 1986; Hakama *et al.*, 1982; Kristofferson, 1979). There is a lack of information for social inequalities in cancer in countries of eastern and southern Europe.

Time trends in social inequalities in cancer

Social class differences in cancer have been remarkably present over time. In specific cancers, however, the magnitude, or even the pattern of the variation by social class has not necessarily been constant throughout the years. As societies change, patterns in health may change. Two of the clearest examples of changes with time of social inequalities in cancer can be seen in Great Britain. In 1950, manual social classes were for the first time recorded having higher lung cancer mortality than non-manual social classes. This was a result of the gradually increasing uptake of smoking by male manual workers, who earlier this century smoked less than males in higher social classes.

In more recent years, a comparison of mortality by social class for lung cancer, ischaemic heart disease and cerebrovascular disease in the periods 1970–72 and 1979–83 showed that despite a general decline in mortality from these causes, differentials between non-manual and manual social classes widened (Marmot and McDowall, 1986) (Figure 3). This was particularly true for women in manual social classes for whom, contrary to patterns for men and for women of non-manual social classes, lung cancer mortality rose during these years. The authors of this report attributed the widening in mortality by social class to widening differences in smoking, together with the effect of other differences in behaviour and also the effect of unemployment and of increased income differentials.

Cancer in the unemployed

Studies on socio-economic status and cancer mainly examine differences among those employed. The health of the unemployed has been studied less although in many societies they constitute a significant part of the population, and may live in conditions of material deprivation worse than those of the lowest social class. Studies on unemployment in the pre-war recession and in recent periods have shown beyond doubt that becoming unemployed is associated with stress-related behaviour, and that those unemployed have worse mental and physical health than those employed. Information, especially from prospective studies, on the health of the unemployed is unfortunately largely lacking.

Cancer incidence and mortality data from the OPCS Longitudinal Study (Moser *et al.*, 1986; Kogevinas, 1990) have shown that those unemployed in 1971 had, during the period 1971–81, around 30% higher overall mortality and similarly about 30% increased cancer incidence compared with those employed. Results from this nationwide study indicated that unemployment, either directly or indirectly, had adversely affected the health of unemployed men; there was only limited support for an hypothesis purporting that increased mortality of the unemployed simply reflected the poorer health of those most likely to become unemployed (ill-health selection hypothesis).

How can social inequalities in cancer be explained?

Even if the molecular basis of carcinogenesis is still largely unknown, many factors causing cancer have been identified, allowing in some instances the implementation of cancer prevention programmes (for a review see IARC, 1990a; IARC, 1990b). One approach therefore to explaining social inequalities in

a) Men aged 20 to 64

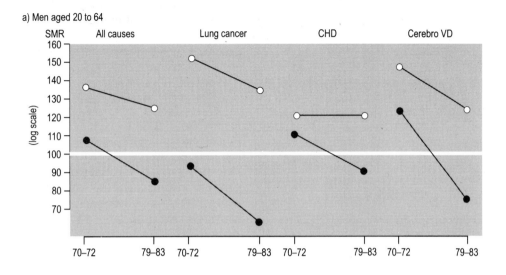

(b) Married women aged 20 to 54 classified by husband's occupation

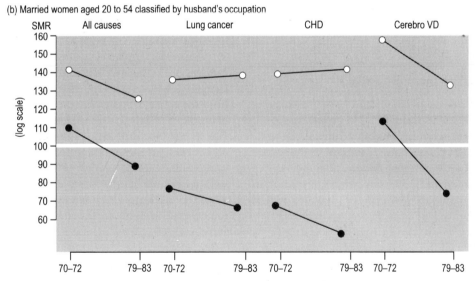

Standardised mortality ratios* for select causes of death in Great Britain 1970–1972 and 1979–1983 for manual (○—○) and non-manual (●—●) groups

*For each cause the SMR in 1979–1983 is 100 for each sex.

Figure 3 Standard mortality rates for select causes of death in Great Britain 1970-72 and 1979-83 for manual and non-manual groups

cancer is to examine the distribution of known causes of cancer among social classes, and then identify how important these risk factors may be for the occurrence of social class differences. Could, for example, the higher incidence of cervical cancer among women of lower social classes be due to more frequent sexually transmitted infections among women in these social strata? And if yes, how much of the difference could be due to these infections? The importance of major identified risk factors for cancers where wide social inequalities are observed is discussed below.

Tobacco consumption is a major risk factor for many diseases including cancers of the lung, oesophagus, larynx, oral cavity, pancreas, bladder, kidney and probably a few other sites. In England and Wales, there have been marked differences by social class in smoking habits. In 1972, 31.5% of professional men (social class I) and 56.7% of skilled manual workers were smokers. The corresponding percentages for women with husbands in these two social classes were 28.9% and 44.9% (OPCS, 1985).

Prevalence of smoking has been decreasing during recent years among all social classes, but the decrease is much steeper in the non-manual social classes. Among social class I, 17% of men and 15% of women were smokers in 1984, compared to 49% for men and 36% for women in social class V. This indicates that there are two to three times more current smokers among the lower social classes than there are in the higher social classes. A national survey of smoking habits in the USA for 1985 indicated a similar pattern; for both sexes there was a higher percentage of smokers among blue-collar than among white-collar workers (Weinkamm and Sterling, 1987).

Part, therefore, of the differences by social class in incidence of and mortality from cancer can be ascribed to tobacco smoking, and especially much of the socio-economic variation in cancers of the oral cavity, oesophagus, larynx and lung. Quantitative estimates about the importance of tobacco smoking in defining social inequalities in cancer are lacking. A study in New Zealand provided such estimates indirectly and indicated that smoking explains a large part (but not all) of the excess cancer mortality among tobacco-related cancers in the manual social classes (Pearce and Howard, 1986).

In many countries in the past, smoking was less frequent among women than among men. The importance of tobacco smoking in defining current social inequalities in cancer in women is therefore less obvious. Smoking patterns in many societies are, however, changing fast, and women are increasingly taking up smoking. This will undoubtedly result in a replication among women of patterns of social inequalities in cancer that are up until today seen predominantly among men.

Occupational risk factors have been estimated to account for approximately 4 to 6% of all cancers in the population of the USA (Doll and Peto, 1981) and similar estimates probably hold for other industrialized countries. It has been pointed out that in males occupational risk factors account for a higher percentage of all cancers, and in male manual workers this percentage may be as high as 12%. In regions with a high concentration of industry, as much as 40% of all lung cancers have been attributed to occupational risk factors (Vineis and Simonato, 1991).

Neoplasms of the lung, bladder, the pleura, the liver, nose and nasal cavity, the skin, and the leukaemias and lymphomas have been associated more frequently than other neoplasms with exposures in the occupational environment (IARC, 1990a). Any list of occupational carcinogens, or of industries in which employment entails a carcinogenic risk, easily reveals that those principally exposed to workplace carcinogens are blue-collar workers. Even if the overall percentage of cancer due to occupational risk factors is about 4% only, there is a concentration of these risk factors in the manual social classes, contributing therefore in a disproportionate way to social inequalities in cancer.

By simply comparing cancer occurrence between the non-manual and manual social classes it is difficult to determine the degree to which elevated cancer mortality is related to occupation, and that to which it is related to general social circumstances. Apart from variation in occupational exposures, social classes differ in many other aspects of life. An analysis of national mortality data from England and Wales showed that both occupation and way of life contributed to the variation in cancer mortality between occupational groups (Fox and Adelstein, 1978).

Among cancers showing large or consistent differentials, breast and cervical cancer are those most related to **reproductive and sexual risk factors**. Breast cancer occurs more frequently among women of higher social class, while the opposite pattern is seen for cervical cancer.

Early age of first full-term pregnancy and high parity, are among the factors associated with reduced breast cancer risk; early age of menarche, late age of menopause, first full-term pregnancy after age 35 and nulliparity have been associated with increased risk (IARC, 1990a). Women in the lower social classes in England and Wales tend to have earlier first full-term pregnancies, bigger families and a lower proportion of nulliparity than women in higher social classes. Data from the OPCS Longitudinal Study showed that in 1971, among women aged less than 60 years, 18% of female owner-occupiers were nulliparous and 7.8% had their first child before the age of 20, compared to 8.2% and 18.1% respectively for council tenants (Kogevinas, 1990). These factors contribute to the observed pattern but, both in England and Wales and in the USA, variation in reproductive factors is probably not sufficient to explain the variation between social classes (Devesa and Diamond, 1980).

Early age of first intercourse and promiscuity of women or of their partners are associated with a high risk of cervical cancer; these factors are directly related to the probability of acquiring sexually transmitted infections. Explanations for the socio-economic pattern in cervical cancer have incriminated sexual history as one possible contributing factor. Differences in sexual habits among social classes are, however, poorly understood and frequently based on erroneous assumptions about behaviour of people in different social classes; the limited existing evidence does not identify distinct patterns (Brown *et al.*, 1984). Which factors contribute to social class differences in cervical cancer remain to be proved.

Among cancers where social inequalities are apparent, **alcohol consumption** is associated with cancers of the oral cavity, oesophagus, larynx and liver. Consumption patterns by social class are not as distinct as for tobacco. In England and Wales, about a quarter of men in the manual social classes were classified in 1975 as heavy drinkers, compared with around 10% of men in non-manual occupations (OPCS, 1984). Women in manual occupations are more likely to abstain or to be occasional drinkers than women in non-manual social classes. The risk of oesophageal and laryngeal cancer has been shown to be very high for persons who both smoke and drink, and in this may lie much of the importance of alcohol in increasing inequalities in cancer among males.

The importance of diet in determining cancer risk cannot be overestimated. **Dietary factors** may cause between 30% and 70% of all cancers, although specific aspects of the association between diet and cancer remain to be clarified. Increased intake of fruits and vegetables is associated with lower risk of several cancers, most notably those of the stomach, colon and lung. Increased fat intake is associated with higher risk for cancers of the colon, breast and prostate. Differences in dietary patterns between social classes have not always been well recorded. In recent

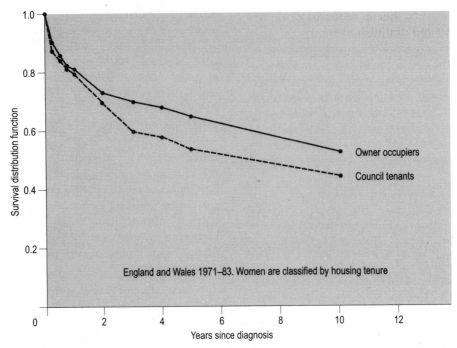

Figure 4 Socio-economic differences in survival among women with cancer of body of the uterus, by year since diagnosis

years, in England and Wales, fresh fruits and vegetables, which probably exert a protective effect for many cancers, are consumed more by those in the higher social classes than in the lower (Cole-Hamilton and Lang, 1986). The importance of diet on social inequalities in cancer has not been estimated.

As mentioned earlier in this paper, social class inequalities in stomach cancer are amongst the widest recorded and reasons for this remain unexplained. Dietary factors are known to be the main causes of stomach cancer, and salty, pickled, and fried foods are believed to exert an adverse effect, while fresh fruits and vegetables exert a protective effect. Better preservation of food through the wider availability of refrigerators, may have contributed to the impressive and consistent decrease in incidence observed in England and Wales and most other countries during the last four or five decades (IARC, 1990a). The extent to which diet, or preservation of food, contributes to the observed social class differences for this cancer is not known.

General explanations

Examining variation in identified risk factors may help us understand specific causes of social inequalities in cancer and direct us in taking specific preventive measures. This is especially true for occupational cancers, as they primarily occur among men and women in the manual social classes. In most other situations, however, in order that an intervention be successful, the social causes of differences in exposure and lifestyle must be kept in mind. For instance, it is not enough to identify smoking as a causal factor in the wide social class differences in the frequency of lung cancer. It is also appropriate to identify reasons why smoking is more prevalent among the lower social classes; or, similarly, to identify reasons why lower social classes are giving up smoking more slowly than the higher social classes.

The identification of intervening variables that contribute to socio-economic differences in cancer may occasionally lead to important public health benefits. In order, however, to understand and diminish inequalities in cancer, it is appropriate to focus on the chain of causation. Social forces lead to lifestyle and exposure differences, which lead to health differences. It is necessary to ask what are the intermediaries between social class and cancer, such as smoking or occupation, but it is also necessary to understand the social forces that cause these differences in the first place.

A second reason for not limiting our understanding of social inequalities in cancer to the identification of intervening factors, such as alcohol and diet, is that those risk factors already identified do not account for all, and for some diseases maybe not even for the major part, of the incidence or mortality differences in health.

Research on general mortality and on health effects other than cancer is of relevance. In the Alameda County Human Population Laboratory in California, people with adequate income had, throughout the period of follow-up, a higher probability of surviving than those with adequate, marginal and inadequate income (Kaplan, 1985). It was reported that with over 18 years of follow-up, those with inadequate family incomes had 2.1 times the risk of death of those with adequate incomes. After taking into account differences between the income groups in age, sex, race, smoking, alcohol consumption, sleep habits, leisure time, physical activity, body mass index and baseline health status, there was still an increased risk of 1.6 for those with adequate income. If all these factors, which are strongly related to all-cause mortality, are taken into account, and there is still a high risk left unexplained, then what could account for the poorer health associated with lower socio-economic position? Similar findings were observed in the Whitehall study, a large British study of civil servants (Marmot et al.,

1978). Quantitative estimates for the effect of known risk factors on social inequalities in cancer are not readily available.

Psycho-social factors have been shown to contribute to the general increase in physical illness among socio-economic groups. Studies on this topic dealing with cancer, however, have not provided evidence as convincing as that from studies in cardiovascular diseases (IARC, 1990a).

The possibility that childhood exposures may affect risk in adult life has mainly been examined through geographic analyses which have identified a correlation between indicators of childhood deprivation and all-cause mortality, mortality from respiratory diseases, and from heart diseases in adulthood; these studies cannot exclude the possibility of adverse social conditions prevailing in adulthood (Marmot et al., 1987; Davey Smith et al., 1990). Less evidence has been found in these studies for the importance of early childhood exposures on adult cancer risk.

Studies on migrants have indicated that stomach cancer probably provides the clearest example, among other major cancers, of the importance of childhood exposures. Risk for this cancer among migrants moving from a high-risk to a low-risk country remains high, similar to that in the country of origin, even after many years of residence in the host country.

In contrast to stomach cancer, risk for other cancers, for example cancer of the colon and rectum, verges on the levels of the host country much earlier, just a few years after migration. This pattern has been observed in various migrating populations and the persistence of the high risk of stomach cancer has been attributed to exposures occurring in early life. A similar mechanism may therefore be envisaged for explaining in part the social inequalities in cancer in adulthood.

Why should we study social inequalities in cancer?

What can the study of social class inequalities tell us about the causation of a disease? Three reasons can be put forward: public health action, research strategy and theory (Marmot *et al.*, 1987). These are not exclusive to each other and are considered each one in turn.

The WHO and many national health and social services have recognized the need to take public health measures for the elimination of social class inequalities. Reductions in cancer mortality have been achieved in many countries but have not always coincided with diminished social inequalities; as in the case of lung cancer in England and Wales, while a decline in mortality was observed for the population as a whole, social inequalities actually widened. There is no room for complacency in initiating programmes for the reduction of social inequalities in cancer.

Epidemiological studies identifying distinct patterns in disease occurrence, such as those between social classes, provide clues for understanding disease causation. Aspects of lifestyle and exposure circumstances that are correlated with socio-economic factors are very diverse and consequently examination of social class differences frequently may not point to one specific causal factor. The wide social inequalities observed for specific cancers have, however, helped corroborate evidence from studies examining specific risk factors, and have also helped examine the extent to which identified risk factors explain adequately the occurrence of a disease. Furthermore, studying social inequalities allows us to better understand the chain of causation for multi-factorial diseases, such as cancer, focusing not only on immediate causes but also on more indirect causal factors. Understanding causation in a wider sense is necessary for implementing prevention programmes in the community.

The division into social classes reflects, and produces, economic, political and cultural differences, all of which may have an impact on health. Traditionally in modern medicine, the focus is on individuals, individual biological make-up and individual choices about lifestyle. This approach to examining health and disease, while not incorrect, is incomplete. Social class inequalities in health, such as the data on cancer presented in this paper, indicate clearly that whatever the individual differences may be, there are broad social forces determining health and disease status. Social class analysis holds therefore the potential for examining the way in which the organization of society affects health and disease.

References

Brown, S., Vessey, M. and Harris, R. (1984) Social class, sexual habits and cancer of the cervix, *Community Med.* **6**, 281–286.

Cole-Hamilton, I. and Lang, T. (1986) *Tightening belts. A report on the impact of poverty on food*, The London Food Commission, LFC Report No. 13, London.

Davey Smith, G., Bartley, M. and Blane, D. (1990) The Black Report on socio-economic inequalities in health 10 years on, *Br. Med J.* **301**, 373–377.

Desplanques, G. (1976) *La mortalité des adultes suivant le milieu social 1955–71* (Collection de l'INSEE No. 195, Série D., No. 44), Institut National de Statistiques et Études Économiques, Paris.

Devesa, S.S. and Diamond, E.L. (1980) Association of breast cancer and cervical cancer incidences with income and education among whites and blacks, *J. Natl. Cancer Inst.* **65**, 515–528.

Doll, R. and Peto, R. (1981) *The causes of cancer*, Oxford University Press, Oxford-New York.

Fox, A.J. and Adelstein, A.M. (1978) Occupational mortality: work or way of life?, *J. Epidemiol. Comm. Hlth.* **32**, 73–78.

Fox, A.J. and Goldblatt, P.O. (1982) *Longitudinal Study: socio-demographic mortality differentials, 1971–1975*, OPCS Series LS No. 1, HMSO London, 1–227.

Hakama, M., Hakulinen, T., Pukkala, E., Saxén, E. and Teppo, L. (1982) Risk indicators of breast and cervical cancer on ecologic and individual levels, *Am. J. Epidemiol.* **16**, 990–1000.

IARC (1990a) *Cancer: causes, occurrence and control*, IARC Scientific Publications Volume 100, International Agency for Research on Cancer, Lyon.

IARC (1990b) *Evaluating effectiveness of primary prevention of cancer.* IARC Scientific Publications Volume 103, International Agency for Research on Cancer, Lyon.

Kaplan, G.A. (1985) *Twenty years of health in Alameda County: the human population laboratory analyses*, Presented at the Annual Meeting of the Society for Prospective Medicine, San Francisco, California.

Kogevinas, M. (1990) *Longitudinal Study 1971–1983. Socio-demographic differences in cancer survival*, OPCS Series LS No. 5, HMSO, London, 1–97.

Kristoffersen, L. (1979) *Occupational Mortality* (Rapporter fra Statistik Sentralbyro 79/19), Statistik Sentralbyro, Oslo.

Logan, W.P.D. (1982) *Cancer mortality by occupation and social class, 1851–1971.* IARC Scientific Publications No. 36, OPCS SMPS No. 44, HMSO, London, 1–252.

Lynge, E. (1979) *Dødelighed og Erhverv, 1970-75* (Statistiske Undersøgelser No. 37), Danmarks Statistik, Copenhagen.

Marmot, M.G., Kogevinas, M. and Elston, M.A. (1987) Social/economic status and disease, *Ann. Rev. Public Hlth.* **8**, 111–135.

Marmot, M.G., McDowall, M.E. (1986) Mortality decline and widening social inequalities, *Lancet* **2**, 274–276.

Marmot, M.G., Rose, G., Shipley, M., Hamilton, P.J.S. (1978) Employment grade and coronary heart disease in British civil servants, *J. Epidemiol. Comm. Hlth.* **32**, 244–249.

Moser, K.A., Fox, A.J., Jones, D.R. and Goldblatt, P.O. (1986) Unemployment and mortality: further evidence from the OPCS Longitudinal Study 1971–1981, *Lancet* **1**, 365–367.

Office of Population Censuses and Surveys (1984) *General household survey 1982*, OPCS, HMSO, London.

Office of Population Censuses and Surveys (1985) *General household survey – cigarette smoking 1972–1984* (GHS 85/2, London, OPCS Monitor).

Pearce, N.E. and Howard, J.K. (1986) Occupational, social class and male cancer mortality in New Zealand, 1974–1978, *Int. J. Epidemiol.* **15**, 456–462.

Vagero, I. and Persson, G. (1986) Occurrence of cancer in socio-economic groups in Sweden. An analysis based on the Swedish Cancer Environment Registry, *Scand. J. Soc. Med.* **14**, 151–160.

Vineis, P. and Simonato, L. (1991) Proportion of lung and bladder cancers in males resulting from occupation: a systematic approach, *Arch. Environ. Hlth.* **46**, 6–15.

Weinkamm, J.J. and Sterling, T.D. (1987) Changes in smoking characteristics by type of employment from 1970 to 1979/80, *Am. J. Ind. Med.* **11**, 539–561.

THE IMPORTANCE OF THE SOCIAL DIMENSIONS OF CANCER

Elsebeth Lynge

Cancer as a life event

There are 730,000 deaths from cancer every year within the European Community, and it was estimated recently that 1,186,000 new cancer cases are diagnosed every year (Jensen *et al.*, 1990). Cancer is thus a social reality which confronts all of us in our everyday life. The Swedish Cancer Society has summarized the message on posters saying 'every third person will be hit'.

The total of 25,000 new cancer cases in Denmark per year (Storm *et al.*, 1990) is reflected in 111,000 hospitalizations with cancer as the main diagnosis (Sundhedsstyrelsen, 1985). But cancer treatment and prevention also covers a broad register of other activities. An example is the 630,000 screenings which are made each year in order to avoid invasive cases of cervical cancer (Sundhedsstyrelsen, 1986). Cancer is thus a heavy burden on our health care system.

Cancer and age

Cancer risk increases rapidly with age. Fewer than 1% of cancer cases occur in persons below the age of 20 years, and almost 50% of cancer cases occur in persons above the age of 70 years (Storm *et al.*, 1990). Age is therefore in itself an important social dimension of cancer.

Age is also a factor which should always be taken into account when cancer is studied across other social dimensions. This can be illustrated by an example. There is the same number of cancer cases in men and women in Denmark. The numbers were 12,243 and 12,749 new cases, respectively, in 1987. Women are, however, on average older than

men, and the cancer risk was in fact higher in men than in women. The age-standardized rates per 100,000 in a World Standard Population were 310 and 289, respectively. The absolute numbers and the age-standardized rates are therefore different indicators of the cancer occurrence. The first is relevant for planning of hospital beds, the second is relevant for evaluation of risks.

An excess cancer risk following exposure to a carcinogenic agent is seen normally only after a latency period of 20 years or more. Cancer cases today therefore reflect living conditions earlier in life.

Cancer incidence in social groups

From the EC countries, cancer incidence data by social groups are available only from England and Wales (Leon, 1987) and from Denmark (Lynge and Thygesen, 1990). Both data sets are follow-up studies of the 1970/71 census populations. The data from England and Wales are based on a 1% sample of the population, representing roughly 500,000 persons. The data from Denmark cover the whole population, representing roughly 5 million persons. The data on the overall cancer incidence by main social groups in England and Wales and in Denmark are shown in Figure 1. The dates are presented as age-standardized incidence ratios.

There is a gradient in the cancer incidence for men from England and Wales from a standardized incidence ratio (SIR) of 85 in social class I (professionals) to an SIR of 106 in social class IV and V (semi-skilled and

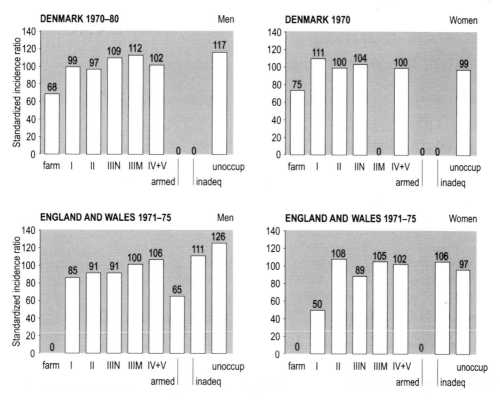

Figure 1   Cancer incidence by social class in England and Wales 1971–75 and in Denmark 1970–80

unskilled workers). This pattern is not so straightforward in Denmark. Social class I has an SIR of 99, and social class IV and V has an SIR of 102. The extremes in Denmark are found for farmers, SIR = 68, and for social class IIIM (skilled workers), where the SIR is 112.

Social history probably plays a role in the differences between the patterns in England and Wales and in Denmark. The transition from an agricultural society to an industrial society was late in Denmark. At least one-quarter of the semi-skilled and unskilled workers in industry in Denmark in 1970 has a background in agriculture. The cancer pattern seen in these workers therefore reflects a life with the first 10 to 20 working years spent in the low-risk agricultural sector and the

following years spent in the high-risk industrial sector.

Unemployed men form a high-risk group for cancer, both in England and Wales and in Denmark. This is notable, because these men were not sick from cancer when they were registered as unemployed in the 1970/71 census. They developed their cancer disease after the census. Unemployed men thus seem to be a particularly vulnerable group for development of cancer.

The cancer incidence data for women show no straightforward gradient over social groups. Unemployed women are primarily housewives and this big group of women has a cancer incidence close to the average.

The social distribution of specific cancer diseases

Cancer is not just one disease. It is a variety of diseases. The number of disease groups that one may distinguish between depends on how detailed the classification is made on sub-site (localization) and cell type (histology). Cancer registry statistics normally distinguish between 40 to 50 cancer diseases defined mainly by localization.

The same classification as the one which is normally used in cancer registry statistics was applied to the Danish follow-up study of the 1970 census population. At the same time, the men who were economically active at the time of the 1970 census were classified into 20 socio-economic groups. Table 1 shows for each cancer site the ratio between the highest and the lowest incidence for these 20 socio-economic groups. The table also shows the cumulative incidence for each cancer site for men below the age of 75 years. The cumulative incidence is an indicator of how frequent the particular cancer type is.

What this table shows is that the widest ranges in the social distribution are found for certain rare cancers with relatively well defined aetiology. The cancer sites with a five-fold or larger range together constitute only 7% of the cumulative cancer incidence. Within this group of cancers we find lip cancer, which is related to sunlight exposure, pleural cancer, which is related to asbestos exposure, and nasal cancer, which is related to wood dust exposure. Cancers of the liver and oesophagus, which are related to alcohol consumption, also have a wide range of incidence, as do cancers of the mouth, larynx and pharynx, which are related to both tobacco and alcohol consumption (Tomatis *et al.*, 1990).

Within the group of cancers with less than a two-fold difference between the socio-economic groups we find some of the more common cancer for which little is known about the aetiology, for example cancer of the prostate, brain and testis.

An equivalent analysis of the variation across social groups for each cancer site is not possible for England and Wales due to the limited number of cancer cases included in the follow-up study of the 1971 census population.

Table 1 Cancer incidence for men by socio-economic group in Denmark, 1970-80

Type of cancer	Ratio between highest and lowest incidence	Cumulative incidence <75 years
Lip (140)	12.2	0.34
Pleura (162.2)	8.4	0.18
Liver (155.0)	6.7	0.41
Mouth (143–144)	6.6	0.24
Nasal cavity (160)	6.2	0.10
Larynx (161)	5.9	0.68
Pharynx (145–148)	5.8	0.30
Mycosis fungoides (205)	5.2	0.02
Esophagus (150)	5.0	0.48
Lung, not primary (163)	4.6	0.01

Lung (162.0, 162.1)	3.9	7.72
Melanoma (190)	3.4	0.75
Pancreas (157)	3.4	1.16
Hodgkin (201)	3.2	0.23
Other, nonspecified (199)	3.1	0.47
Bone (196)	3.1	0.06
Small intestine (152)	3.1	0.10
Breast (170)	3.0	0.05
Metastases (198)	3.0	0.53
Tongue (141)	2.9	0.13
Salivary glands (142)	2.8	0.07
Multiple myeloma (203)	2.8	0.34
Mediastinum (164)	2.7	0.04
Bladder (181)	2.5	2.90
Peritoneum (158–159)	2.4	0.12
Kidney (180)	2.3	1.20
Colon (153)	2.3	2.44
Connective tissue (197)	2.3	0.09
Other genital (179)	2.3	0.11
Other skin (191)	2.3	4.95
Endocrine glands (195)	2.3	0.06
Liver, not primary (156)	2.0	0.20
Gallbladder (155.1)	1.9	0.23
Eye (192)	1.9	0.10
Thyroid (194)	1.9	0.10
Prostate (177)	1.9	3.14
Testis (178)	1.9	0.65
Brain (193)	1.9	1.02
Rectum (154)	1.8	1.82
Non-Hodgkin's lymphoma (200, 202)	1.7	0.70
Leukemia (204)	1.5	0.99
All cancer	1.9	36.68

Source: Lynge and Thygesen, 1990

The social gradient is not uniform

The social class gradient in overall mortality as found in the Decennial Supplements on Occupational Mortality has always shown a low mortality in the economically and educationally advantaged social class I, and a high mortality in the disadvantaged social class V (OPCS, 1986).

The social distribution of different cancer diseases is, however, not uniform. Figure 2 shows the social distribution for men in Denmark for the most common cancers, i.e. the cancers with the highest cumulative incidence.

Stomach cancer was the most common cancer in men when cancer registration started in Denmark in 1943. Since then the disease has been on the decline in many other developed countries as well (Storm *et al.*, 1990). Figure 2 indicates that academics seem to be ahead of other men in this development.

Cancers of the lung, bladder and pancreas are all diseases related to smoking. The more than three-fold difference between the lung cancer

incidence in Danish farmers and the lung cancer incidence in Danish building workers is, however, probably not explained only by differences in smoking. Occupational exposures such as asbestos, silica dust, coal-tar pitches and work as a painter are associated with an increased lung cancer risk (Tomatis *et al.*, 1990). These exposures are all relevant for skilled building workers.

Academics or professionals are at high risk for cancer of the colon and kidney, and to some extent also for cancer of the brain and prostate. Highly suspected risk factors for colon cancer are consumption of red meat (Willett *et al.*, 1990) and sedentary work (Littlemore *et al.*, 1990). A known risk factor for kidney cancer is analgesic mixtures containing phenacetin (Tomatis *et al.*, 1990). The aetiology is, however, in general not well known for these cancers which occur in excess risks among well-educated men.

Academics also have an excess risk of non-melanoma skin cancer. Although free health care is provided for everybody in Denmark, a diagnostic bias cannot be excluded as an explanation for the high risk of these non-lethal cancer lesions among academics.

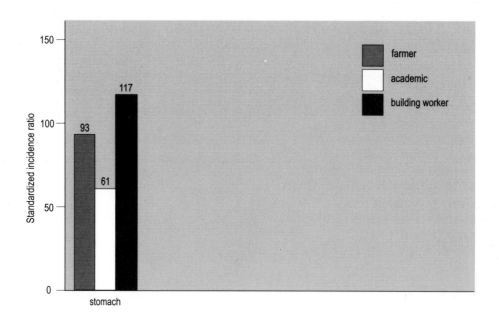

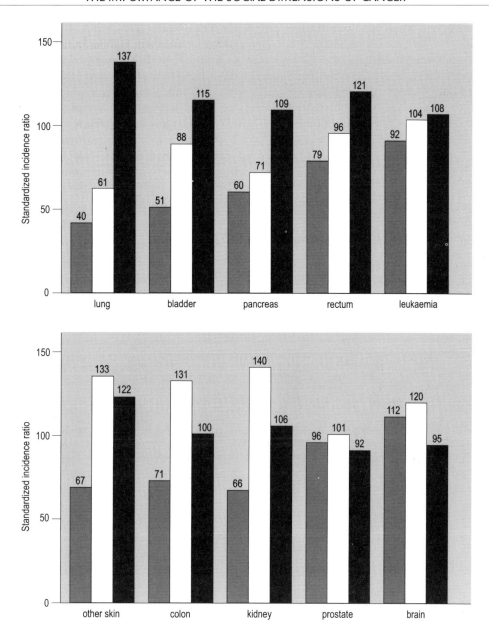

Figure 2 Cancer incidence for selected socio-economic groups of men in Denmark 1970–80

There is a very steep social gradient for women in both lung cancer and cervical cancer, as shown in Figure 3. Cervical cancer is related to sexual habits and the risk increases with increasing number of sexual partners. This risk is suspected to be associated with viral infections, primarily human papilloma virus and herpes simplex virus (Tomatis *et al.*, 1990).

There is also a steep social gradient in breast cancer and uterine corpus cancer. The gradient here goes, however, in the opposite direction to the one found for cancer of the lung and cervix.

Parity and early age at first birth are known to protect against the risk of breast cancer (Tomatis *et al.*, 1990). Later births might contribute to the increased breast cancer risk in academics. Oestrogen replacement therapy increases the risk of cancer of the uterine corpus as does obesity (Tomatis *et al.*, 1990) Intermittent sunlight exposure, as one may experience during vacations in hot areas, increases the risk of malignant melanomas (Tomatis *et al.*, 1990). The higher melanoma occurrence in academics may thus reflect a greater access to recreational activities, especially in their childhood.

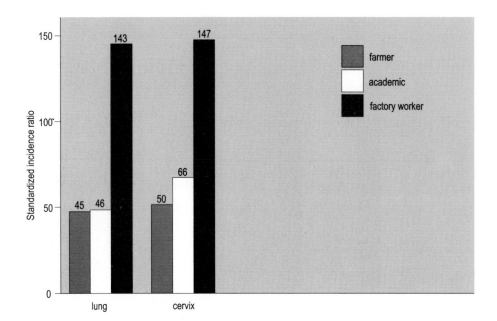

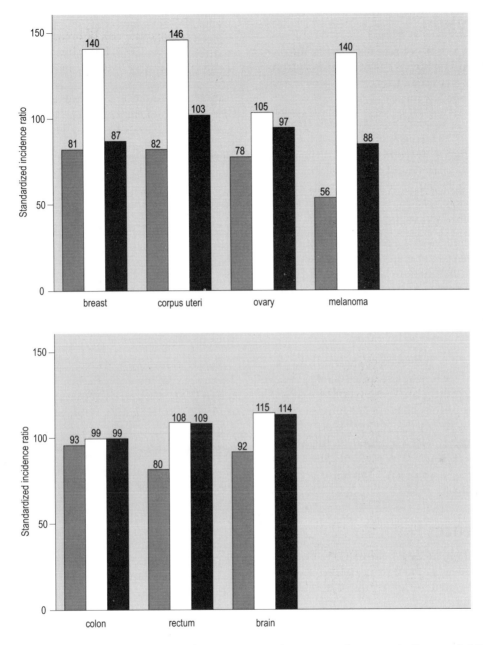

Figure 3 Cancer incidence for selected socio-economic groups of women in Denmark 1970–80

Conclusion

Cancer is a common disease. 'Every third person will be hit.' What we can learn from the social pattern of cancer is, however, that we are not all at the same risk.

If the entire Danish population had the same cancer risk as farmers, one-third of the cancer cases in males, and one-quarter of the cancer cases in women would not occur. This is intriguing, because the way of farm life, which is the background for these low cancer figures, is now rapidly disappearing.

The differences in the social distributions across the spectrum of cancer diseases also point to differences in aetiology. Much has been learned about the carcinogenic risk from smoking and work-place exposures by studying the cancers at high risk among skilled and unskilled workers.

Our society is, however, changing from an industrial society to a service society. The well educated groups are those who have lived the life of a service society for the longest period. Important knowledge about the possible future cancer risks from modern life may therefore be learned by studying the cancers now in excess among academics and professionals.

References

Jensen, O.M., Estève, J., Møller, H., Bonard, H. (1990) Cancer in the European Community and its member states, *Eur. J. Cancer* **26**, 1167–1256.

Leon, D.A. (1987) *Longitudinal study. Social distribution of cancer*. Office of Population Censuses and Surveys. Series LS no. 3, HMSO, London.

Lynge, E., Thygesen, L. (1990) Occupational cancer in Denmark. Cancer incidence in the 1970 census population, *Scand. J. Work Environ. Hlth.* **16**, (suppl 2), 1–35.

Office of Population Censuses and Surveys (1990) *Occupational mortality. Part I Commentary*, Series DS no. 6, HMSO, London.

Storm, H.H., Manders, T., Sprøgel, P., Bang, S., Jensen, O.M. (1990) *Cancer incidence in Denmark 1987*, Danish Cancer Society. Danish Cancer Registry, Copenhagen.

Sundhedsstyrelsen (1985) *Use of hospital beds 1985*, Sygehusstatistik II, 34, Copenhagen, (in Danish).

Sundhedsstyrelsen (1986) Mass screening for cervical cancer. Underudvalget Vedrørende livmoderhalskræftundersøqelse, Copenhagen, (in Danish).

Tomatis, L., Aitio, A., Day, N.E., Heseltine, E., Kaldor, J., Miller, A.B., Parkin, D.M., Riboli, E. (eds.) (1990) *Cancer: causes, occurrence and control*, IARC Scientific Publications No. 100, Lyon.

Willett, W.C., Stampfer, M.J., Colditz, G.A., Rosner, B.A., Speizer, F.E. (1990) Relation of meat, fat and fibre intake to the risk of colon cancer in a prospective study among women, *N. Engl. J. Med.* **323**, 1664–1672.

Wittemore, A.S., Wu-Williams, A.H., Lee, M., Shu, Z., Gallagher, R.P., Deng-ao, J., Lun Z., Xianghui, W., Kun, C., Jung, D., Teh C.Z., Chengde, L., Yao, X.J., Paffenbarger, R.S., Henderson, B.E. (1990) Diet, physical activity and colorectal cancer among Chinese in North America and China, *J. Natl. Cancer Inst.* **82**, 915–926.

CLINICAL TRIALS IN CANCER PREVENTION

Marc Buyse, Philippe Autier and Pascal Piedbois

The goal of prevention studies

Preventive interventions aiming to reduce the incidence of some cancers involve either removing a risk factor (e.g. asbestos or benzenic compounds) or introducing a preventive measure (e.g. encouraging smokers to quit smoking).

The goal of prevention studies of cancer is to evaluate the possible impact of an intervention on a given cancer (or on all cancers). This evaluation requires one to demonstrate that there is a difference between two similar groups of subjects, one given the intervention and the other not. 'Similarity' of the groups of subjects implies that the risk factors for the disease to be prevented are evenly distributed between both groups. If a risk factor were not evenly distributed between the groups, then the influence of that risk factor might confound any effect of the intervention. For instance, in a study on the prevention of colorectal cancer by high fibre intake, two groups of subjects would be compared: one with diet rich in fibre and one with their usual diet. If the group with high fibre intake happened by chance to include a higher percentage of people with a familial history of colorectal cancer, then the study might very well fail to demonstrate a possible benefit of high fibre intake.

Experimental vs. non-experimental studies

The first step towards identifying a worthwhile intervention is to review all available evidence supporting it. Such evidence generally comes from both basic research and epidemiology, but it is rarely so overwhelming that it does not need to be confirmed through some kind of prospective experiment. For instance, a thorough review of observational epidemiological studies recently gave support to the hypothesis that a diet rich in fibre may protect against colon cancer (Trock *et al.*, 1990). The outcome of retrospective reviews, however, is to generate plausible hypotheses rather than to provide definitive answers.

When a preventive hypothesis is deemed plausible, prospective studies must be mounted to test it. For instance, a prospective study was conducted among 88,751 female nurses who were asked to complete a dietary questionnaire. A comparison of dietary patterns among the women who developed a colon cancer and those who did not revealed that a high intake of animal fat may increase the risk of colon cancer (Willett *et al.*, 1990). The retrospective review as well as this prospective study are non-experimental, in that there is no attempt to modify the risk factors under study. In some cases, evidence may also come from 'quasi-experimental' studies, i.e. studies in which a risk factor is removed in an uncontrolled fashion. The declining incidence of lung cancer noted after a decrease in cigarette consumption provides a good example of a quasi-experimental setting (Lopez, 1990).

Even though experimental studies that are not truly experimental may provide worthwhile data, they suffer from many weaknesses in demonstrating the impact of a preventive intervention. A decrease in the incidence of a given cancer may be due to a cause other than the decline in the prevalence of the risk factor (e.g. the striking decrease in incidence of gastric cancer is not explained by the removal or attenuation of a known risk factor). It is difficult, in observational studies, to control for risk factors other than those under study. Hence, whenever possible, experimental studies should be organized to confirm the causality and measure the impact of an intervention.

Fundamentals of randomized clinical trials

The need for randomization

Randomization consists of assigning a treatment or some other intervention to subjects or groups of subjects using a change procedure.

The major benefit of randomization is to provide comparability of the randomized groups with respect to all known and unknown factors, thus permitting an unbiased comparison of the groups. No other approach offers the same guarantee against bias. For instance, to evaluate the worth of some preventive intervention, one could think of submitting all eligible subjects to the intervention and then comparing their outcome to historical figures. Such a comparison would almost surely be biased by systematic differences caused by changes over time in the disease incidence, in diagnostic procedures, and in treatment and supportive care.

The trial protocol and committees

As emphasized in other sections of this paper, prevention trials in cancer require extensive resource over long periods of time. Such major undertakings need to be carefully designed and reviewed before they are activated. The first step towards designing a prevention trial is to develop a protocol, as summarized in Table 1. Before the trial is activated, its protocol needs to be seen by an independent Protocol Review Committee which critically reviews its scientific merit as well as its technical aspects. After approval by this Committee, the protocol needs to be approved in each country (or institution) in which it will be conducted by an Ethical Review Committee. While the trial is ongoing, it is usually monitored by a Data Monitoring Committee which evaluates differences emerging in favour of (or against) the preventive intervention, and recommends trial termination if these differences cannot

plausibly be ascribed to change (Steering Committee of the Physicians' Health Study Research Group, 1988).

Table 1 Protocol contents

1	Title page
2	Rationale and scientific background
3	Objectives of the trial
4	Selection of subjects or units
5	Trial design
6	Preventive intervention
7	Follow-up procedures
8	End-points and evaluation criteria
9	Recruitment and randomization of subjects or units
10	Study logistics and data collection
11	Statistical considerations and data analysis
12	Dissemination of results and publication
13	Ethical considerations
14	References

Objectives of prevention trials

Primary prevention is aimed at protecting healthy subjects from getting the disease. The objective of a primary prevention trial is to reduce the incidence of the disease (and thus, ultimately, to reduce the disease-specific mortality).

Common sense dictates that primary prevention is preferable to other forms of interventions, for avoiding a serious disease is certainly wiser than having to treat it! The problem is, of course, that causal factors must be known for the disease to be preventable. Diseases of known aetiology can be, and have been, effectively prevented; for instance, the prevention of smallpox has been so effective that this disease is thought to have been eradicated (no new case has been reported over the last 10 years). Diseases of unknown and/or complex aetiology, such as most cancers, are tremendously difficult to prevent. A first difficulty is that several factors usually need to act together before a cancer develops. The exact role of each factor, and the interaction between them, is in most cases unclear. A second difficulty is that even when risk factors are known, the long-term effects of preventive measures may remain difficult to predict. A last difficulty, perhaps the most troublesome one, is that many factors that are known to cause cancer are an intrinsic part of our lifestyle, such as dietary habits, and are therefore hard to affect.

End-points of prevention trials

Incidence vs. mortality

The most appropriate end-point of primary prevention trials is reduced cancer incidence. The ultimate goal of cancer prevention is to reduce mortality, but mortality may not be a good end-point to monitor for two main reasons. First, death from cancer occurs much later than the disease itself, so that much longer observation times would be needed to detect a real benefit if mortality were the end-point rather than incidence. Second, mortality from other causes generally dominates mortality from the cancer of interest, so any real benefit of the intervention might be obscured by the overall mortality.

Competing risks

The net benefit of an intervention must be measured with respect to all its expected and unexpected effects. For instance, the administration of tamoxifen to women at high risk of breast cancer should not be evaluated only with respect to incidence of (or cause-specific mortality from) breast cancer. It is quite possible that tamoxifen, through its cholesterol-lowering effect, might reduce the incidence of heart disease to a much larger

extent than it would reduce the incidence of breast cancer. On the negative side, it is also possible that tamoxifen, given over long periods of time, might cause an elevation of endometrial cancer (Prentice, 1990). Hence, in a trial of preventive tamoxifen, it would be sensible to follow not only the incidence of breast cancer, but also the incidence of (and mortality from) other diseases, including myocardial infarction and non-breast cancers (see Chemoprevention).

Intermediate end-points

Because of the long latency period in the development of most cancers, any beneficial effect on incidence (and on mortality) will become noticeable only after a considerable period of time. It would be advantageous to study intermediate end-points which occur earlier in the disease process, when such end-points are available. These could include the appearance of pre-cancerous lesions (e.g. colorectal polyps that often precede colorectal cancers) or a change in some biological marker (e.g. an oncogene known to be expressed in the cancer of interest). Valid candidates as intermediate end-points must be causally related to the cancer of interest, and there must be some evidence that they will be affected by the intervention under study.

Design issues in prevention trials

Group randomization

In therapeutic trials, individual patients are assigned randomly between two or more treatments. In prevention trials, it is often preferable to take groups of subjects rather than individuals as the basic units for assigning randomly. The groups can be general practices, hospitals, geographical communities, factories, schools or religious groups (Byar and Freedman, 1990). Group randomization is often chosen for administrative convenience: it is easier to give the intervention to all subjects within a group, rather than to some of them (Alexander et al., 1989). More importantly, the subjects of a group are likely to exchange information, thereby possibly causing some 'contamination' of the intervention. Contamination is especially likely to happen for interventions aimed at altering lifestyles, such as diet modifications or smoking cessation programmes. For some interventions, such as mass education programmes, group randomization may be the only feasible option. Other reasons for group randomization include cost and political considerations (Byar and Freedman, 1990).

Stratification

The Edinburgh randomized trial of breast cancer screening provides an example of group randomization which may serve to introduce the notion of stratification (Alexander *et al.*, 1989). Eighty-seven general practices were chosen at random. The patients of 43 of these general practices were systematically offered mammographic screening, while the patients of the 44 remaining general practices were not.

An analysis of overall mortality in this trial was recently presented (Alexander *et al.*, 1989). In this analysis, the authors observed that the two groups were not well balanced in terms of socio-economic status. The group receiving screening contained more women of higher socio-economic status than the control group. The analysis also showed a higher mortality rate among women of lower socio-economic status. Thus the imbalance between the two groups in terms of socio-economic status may have confounded the effect of screening.

In order to safeguard against such accidental imbalances, it is desirable to 'stratify' the randomization so that the two groups are well balanced with respect to the important prognostic factors. In the Edinburgh trial, the randomization had only been stratified by the number of patients in each practice so as to have about the same number of patients in the screening and in the control groups.

Feasibility studies

Feasibility studies are often needed before large-scale prevention trials are carried out because of the cost and complexity of these trials. The goals of feasibility studies can be to estimate the optimum dosage of a chemopreventive agent, to study subject compliance, to evaluate the feasibility of recruiting large numbers of subjects, or to re-assess the sample size required and trial duration (Greenwald *et al.*, 1990). The duration of feasibility studies can vary from six months to several years (Byar and Freedman, 1990).

Run-in periods

It is often useful, in prevention trials, to allow for a 'run-in' period to assess the compliance of subjects before their inclusion in the trial. During the run-in period, all subjects are submitted to the intervention just as they would be if they were in the intervention group. The subjects whose compliance is unsatisfactory should not be included in the trial, since their low compliance would dilute any true benefit of the intervention (Byar and Freedman, 1990). A trial with a run-in period to reject these subjects will have higher statistical power for the same sample size than a trial without a run-in period. For example, in the US Physicians' Health Study, 33,211 physicians were enrolled in a run-in period, during which they took active aspirin and beta-carotene placebo (Buring and Hennekens, 1989). After 18 weeks, about one-third of the enrolled subjects had an inadequate compliance. These subjects were not randomized in the trial.

The major problem with a run-in period is that the trial itself is then restricted to a group of proven good compliers, resulting in difficulties in generalizing its results to the population as a whole. In short, the results of a trial with a run-in period are likely to be more valid but less readily generalizable.

Factorial designs and interactions

Factorial designs allow one to test two or more physicians in a single trial. They can often be used in prevention trials because the toxicity and side-effects of the intervention are low enough that several interventions can be administered simultaneously.

Consider two interventions, I1 and I2. Each of them can be administered or not. The '2 × 2' factorial design consists of four groups of subjects receiving either I1 and I2 together or at the same doses as when given separately (Freedman and Green, 1990). Distinct analyses can be contemplated to address the following questions about I1: 'What is the overall effect of I1?', 'What is the effect of I1 when I2 is not administered?', and 'What is the effect of I1 when I2 is administered?', and likewise for I2. One potential problem with a factorial design is the possibility of an interaction between I1 and I2. There is a negative interaction between I1 and I2 if the effect of I1 is larger when given with I2 than when given alone. The presence of an interaction, either negative or positive, does in no way invalidate a factorial design, but it may make the results of the trial more difficult to interpret. A negative interaction between I1 and I2 would decrease the power of the trial to detect the effect of either I1 or I2. On the other hand, a positive interaction would increase the power of the trial to detect the effect of either I1 or I2.

The US Physicians' Health Study is an example of prevention trial using a 2 × 2 factorial design (Buring and Hennekens, 1989). The aim of the trial was the simultaneous assessment of the effect of aspirin on cardiovascular mortality, and of the effect of beta-carotene on cancer incidence. An interaction between aspirin and beta-carotene was considered unlikely. Twenty-two thousand physicians were randomized in 4 groups: aspirin placebo plus beta-carotene, and aspirin plus beta-carotene (see Figure 1).

This trial allows two main analyses to be performed: first, a comparison of cardiovascular mortality among the 11,000 physicians taking aspirin compared with the 11,000 not taking it, and second, a comparison of cancer incidence among the 11,000 physicians taking beta-carotene with the 11,000 not taking it (see Figure 2). As a matter of fact, an interim analysis showed a significant reduction in myocardial infarctions among physicians taking aspirin, and this promoted termination of the aspirin component of the study (Steering Committee of the Physicians' Health Study Research Group, 1988). The beta-carotene component of the study is still ongoing.

The major benefit of factorial designs is to avoid multiple, expensive trials by testing two (or more) hypotheses 'for the price of one'. Often a less mature hypothesis (such as beta-carotene for the prevention of cancer) can be a factor in a trial testing a more mature hypothesis (such as aspirin for the prevention of myocardial infarction). The sample sizes need not be equal for both questions: in a trial testing a main hypothesis, one could randomize a subgroup of subjects to test a secondary hypothesis. Factorial designs are also particularly appropriate when, in practice, two interventions are likely to be used together. Conducting two separate trials in such a situation would be less realistic, and would lead to less generalizable results (Freedman and Green, 1990).

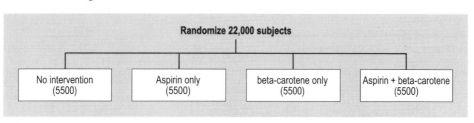

Figure 1 Randomization in a 2 × 2 factorial design

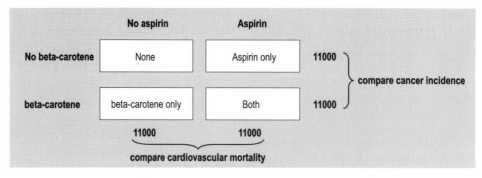

Figure 2 Analysis of a 2 × 2 factorial design

Blinding and placebos

'Double-blinded' randomized trials, in which neither the patient nor the physician knows which drug is delivered, are considered an ideal design to eliminate bias in the assessment of treatment results. They are, however, rarely feasible in therapeutic cancer trials, because of the acute toxicity of most cancer treatments. 'Placebo-controlled' randomized trials, in which the patients of one group receive an inactive substance identical in taste and appearance to the active drug, are also rarely performed in cancer treatment trials due to the need to offer an active treatment to all patients.

Unlike in cancer treatment trials, blinding and the use of a placebo are desirable features in cancer prevention trials, particularly in chemoprevention trials. The use of a placebo group rather than an untreated control group may greatly reduce contamination of the intervention by 'drop-ins'. For instance, the US Physicians' Health Study of aspirin and beta-carotene was conducted as a placebo-controlled trial. Another example is a trial aimed at evaluating retinoids to reduce the risk of skin cancer: subjects with a history of at least ten actinic keratoses were randomized to receive either retinol or a placebo (Moon, 1989).

Avoidance of contamination

There is 'contamination' in a prevention trial when subjects randomized to one of the groups follow the recommendations of, or take the

agent prescribed in, the other group. Imagine two individuals randomized in a prevention trial, one in the intervention group, the other one in the control group. If these individuals work in the same company, or live in the same neighbourhood, they may exchange information on the intervention, and there is a serious risk of contamination. Contamination is a problem in so far as it reduces the difference between the intervention group and the control group, thereby weakening the likelihood that the trial will detect a true effect of the intervention.

It is important to consider the possibility of contamination in the sample size calculation (Moon, 1989). As stated above, group randomization can substantially reduce the risk of contamination. Nevertheless, for lifestyle interventions (e.g. dietary modifications), increasing the awareness of the general population about the intervention is possible, and its impact on both the control and the intervention groups must be estimated before the trial is initiated.

An extreme form of contamination is created by subjects who do not stay at all in the group they were allocated to by the randomization. 'Drop-outs' are subjects who were initially allocated to the intervention and decided to quit it. 'Drop-ins' are subjects who were initially allocated to the control group, but decided to adopt the intervention. Drop-outs are more likely in a prevention trial than in a treatment trial, because of the longer duration of a prevention trial and because the motivation of patients randomized in a treatment trial is usually higher.

Measurement of exposure

The measurement of exposure to the intervention, or of the subject compliance to the intervention, is required for a proper interpretation of the trial results. Subjective methods of measurement may be as simple as asking questions to the subjects (Moon 1989). In drug-based prevention trials, it is possible (though far from satisfactory) to count the number of pills returned by the subjects at each follow-up visit. Objective measurements of exposure through biological markers, when they exist and can realistically be used, are far more reliable. Examples are the urinary excretion of nicotine in subjects who are supposed to give up smoking, or the blood levels of beta-carotene in subjects who are supposed to take beta-carotene supplements (Greenwald *et al.*, 1990).

The preventive intervention

Mode of action and nature of intervention

Human cancers result from multiple changes in cellular genetic material. It is classical, even if possibly oversimplified, to divide the carcinogenetic process into two phases: the initiation phase and the promotion phase. At the heart of the carcinogenetic process is the activation of proto-oncogenes into oncogenes through various mechanisms, including exposure to chemical carcinogens. The carcinogenetic process is followed by a pre-clinical period, during which the subject is not aware that a cancer is present (see Figure 3). This period may vary from five to 15 years.

Interventions to prevent cancer can take place at different stages in the carcinogenetic process. Some interventions aim at preventing the initiation phase of the carcinogenetic process. Such interventions require very long follow-up times to be evaluated, since a reduction in the incidence of cancer can only be seen after a period at least equal to the duration of the carcinogenetic phase plus that of the pre-clinical period. Other interventions are thought to affect the promotion phase of the carcinogenetic process. The observation times needed to observe their possible benefits are shorter, but the interpretation of observed patterns in cancer incidence after such interventions is far from straightforward (Zelen, 1988).

Interventions can be classified more specifically according to their mode of action. The intervention can be based on the suppression of the exposure to a chemical carcinogen. Smoking cessation and dietary modifications to reduce the amount of animal fat and of smoked food are examples of this class of exposure-based interventions. Another class of interventions is based on the inactivation or the excretion of carcinogens before they may have an action. Antioxidants such as Vitamins C or E, through their theoretical ability to prevent the formation of nitrosamines in the digestive tract, and dietary modifications to increase the intake of fibres, are examples of this class. A third class of interventions is based on either the inhibition of proto-oncogene activation, or the blockage of their expression (Greenwald *et al.*, 1990). Tumour-suppressive retinoids and steroid hormones are agents of this class.

Another way of classifying the various interventions is by their nature: drugs or dietary supplements, dietary modifications, or lifestyle (behavioural) modifications. Examples of each of these are shown in Table 2 and are further discussed in the sections on Lifestyle Modifications through to Chemoprevention.

Table 2 Some of the many possible preventive interventions, by cancer site and type of intervention

Cancer	Intervention	Type
All cancers	beta-carotene	Drug
Basal cell	isotretinoin	Drug
Breast	reduction in fat intake	Diet
	4-hydroxyphenyl retinamide	Drug
	tamoxifen	Drug
Colorectal	increase in fibre intake	Diet
	reduction in animal fat intake	Diet
Oesophagus	multi-vitamin supplements	Drug
Lung	smoking cessation	Lifestyle
	beta-carotene	Drug
	alpha-tocopherol	Drug
Melanoma	reduction in UV exposure	Lifestyle
Stomach	reduction in salt-cured and smoked food	Diet

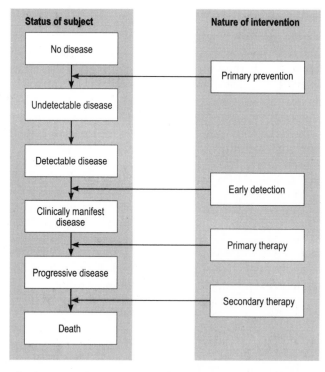

Figure 3 Interventions at successive stages in the disease process

Lifestyle modifications

Prevention trials based on lifestyle modifications are the most difficult to undertake. When the benefit of the suppression of a carcinogen is clear, as it is for smoking cessation, the end-point of the trial is not the reduction in cancer incidence or mortality, but the effectiveness of the programme. Smoking is responsible for about 30% of all cancer deaths throughout Europe, and there is little question that a reduction in smoking does translate directly into a reduction in cancer incidence.

In the Community Intervention Trial (COMMIT), for instance, 22 communities were divided randomly into two groups, one group receiving interventions aimed at smoking cessation, the other group being used as a control. The interventions involved health-care providers, work-sites, organizations, smoking cessation resources and services, public education, and schools. This is the largest smoking intervention study in the world, involving two million people directly. The 11 pairs of communities were matched for size, demographics, and location. The study was designed to detect a 10% difference in the smoking quit rate between the two groups (Freedman and Green, 1990).

Quite apart from the enormous logistical difficulties in such exposure-based prevention trials, their application is limited because for the majority of cancers, a physical or chemical aetiologic factor has not been identified (Greenwald et al., 1990).

Dietary modifications

Prevention trials based on dietary modifications may be somewhat easier to conduct than those based on lifestyle modifications. For example, strong evidence exists which shows that the risk of colon cancer is correlated with dietary fat, particularly from animal sources (Willett et al., 1990). Dietary fibres, conversely, may reduce this risk (Trock et al., 1990). A randomized prevention trial, comparing a reduction in

animal fat intake with a control group, would provide stronger evidence on the possibility of reducing the risk of colon cancer through modifications of dietary patterns than observational studies.

But such a trial would present various difficulties. First, dietary habits may prove difficult to change in the intervention group. The risk of drop-outs (subjects in the intervention group who quit it) would be high because of the long duration of the trial. Second, secular trends in dietary patterns, affecting both the intervention and the control group, might reduce the differences between both groups. The risk of drop-ins (subjects in the control group who effectively join in the intervention) would be high because of the publicity around the recommended dietary changes. Third, the measurement of compliance would be difficult unless biological markers for the dietary intake of specific nutrients were available.

Are such trials feasible? There are two comparable ongoing trials for breast cancer prevention (Self et al., 1988, Boyd et al., 1990). Experimental data have shown that dietary fat intake increases the risk of breast cancer. Epidemiological studies are consistent with the experimental evidence: variations in breast cancer rates between countries are strongly correlated with international variations in estimated dietary fat intake (Boyd et al., 1990). However, a prospective observational study did not show any association between dietary fat intake and breast cancer risk (Willett et al., 1990). In fact, the range of dietary fat intake in western countries may be too narrow to permit the detection of such an association.

This difficulty is circumvented in the randomized trials, in which the range of fat intake can be widely increased. In one of the two ongoing trials, women with extensive mammographic dysplasia are divided randomly into two groups: an intervention group in which dietary fat intake is reduced to a target of 15% of total calories, or a control group receiving dietary advice but without any target for the reduction of dietary fat intake (Boyd *et al.*, 1990). To date, some 600 women have enrolled. At two years, in the intervention group, 60% of the subjects consume less than 20% of calories from fat and 80% consume less than 25% of calories from fat. In the other trial, the target dietary fat intake is 20% of total calories and the target polyunsaturated fat, monounsaturated fat, saturated fat ratio is 1:1:1 (Self *et al.*, 1988).

Chemoprevention

Chemoprevention trials (drug-based prevention trials) are the easiest to conduct. In contrast to the above interventions, the identification of a risk factor or carcinogen is not necessary for a drug to be tested for its preventive efficacy. At present, the US National Cancer Institute (NCI) is sponsoring more than 20 chemoprevention trials (Greenwald *et al.*, 1990). Most of them study vitamins and micronutrient dietary supplements as preventive factors.

An illustrative chemoprevention trial currently under discussion both in the US and in Europe is that of tamoxifen to prevent breast cancer in high-risk women.

A chemoprevention trial has been proposed by the NCI to evaluate the preventive effect of tamoxifen. The trial will enrol 15,000 women aged between 45 and 65 years who are at high risk of developing breast cancer. Individual women will be placed at random into two groups, one group receiving 20 mg tamoxifen a day for 5 years and the other group a placebo. The primary end-points will be incidence of breast cancer and mortality. Patients from both groups will have an annual mammography screening for 10 years. Myocardial infarction will be a secondary end-point, because tamoxifen has been found to reduce LDL-cholesterol, suggesting that it could have a major preventive impact on coronary heart disease (Powles *et al.*, 1989). Other secondary end-points will be studied: other cancers, thromboembolic events, fractures, liver disease and retinopathies.

Of great concern in this trial is the possibly harmful long-term effects of tamoxifen. Tamoxifen has been shown to stimulate the growth of endometrial cancer cells *in vitro* (Anzai *et al.*, 1989), and *in vivo* in the athymic mouse (Gottardis *et al.*, 1988). Tamoxifen has also been shown to act estrogenically by its receptor action (Boccardo *et al.*, 1984), and estrogens can stimulate endometrial carcinogenesis (Ziehl and Finkle, 1975; Smith *et al.*, 1975).

Clinical reports of endometrial cancer after treatment with tamoxifen seem to support the hypothesis of an elevated risk caused by tamoxifen. However, as is often the case, these clinical reports vary greatly in their reliability. Some of them were change observations (Killacke *et al.*, 1985). Some others were reported systematically in a cancer registry, and the possible role of tamoxifen was confirmed through a case-control study (Hardell, 1990). Still others were noted in randomized adjuvant trials using a dose of 40 mg a day of tamoxifen (Fornander, 1989).

In further randomized trials, however, tamoxifen used at a dose of 20 mg a day did not seem to cause any excess risk of endometrial cancer (Ribeiro *et al.*, 1988, Nolvadex Adjuvant Trial Organization, 1988). In view of the potential benefit of tamoxifen given as a preventive agent, and given the conflicting data about its possible adverse effects, random trials are scientifically needed and ethically required to provide a reliable answer to the question of whether tamoxifen can substantially reduce the risk of breast cancer, at least in high-risk subjects.

Target population

General population

Who should be asked to participate in a clinical trial on cancer prevention? A first approach might be to offer participation to subjects from the general population who are within the age range in which cancer is most likely to develop. Should a trial with such subjects show a benefit from the intervention, its conclusions would be readily applicable to the general population.

Yet conducting a prevention trial in the general population presents a number of problems. First, the people who agree to participate in the trial and who are good compliers are usually at lower risk of developing the disease under study. As a consequence, the incidence rate of the cancer of interest is often lower among the trial subjects than among the general population, and this may have a serious negative impact on the power of the trial. Second, compliance may be lower among the general population, which is at low risk of developing the cancer of interest, than among groups of individuals who know they are at higher than normal risk. Third, many cancers have a low incidence rate, and enormous sample sizes are needed to study the effects of a preventive measure on their incidence (see the section on Sample Size Calculations).

High-risk groups

To circumvent the problems of a general population approach, the current tendency is to focus on subjects at elevated risk of developing the cancer of interest. For instance, to study the prevention of colorectal cancer, one may restrict the trial to subjects of 53 years old or more who have a first degree relative with a colorectal cancer or who have been found to have several adenomatous polyps in their large bowel. As stated above, the main motivation for restricting one's attention to high-risk groups is that more end-points will tend to be observed among high-risk subjects, and thus for the same number of enrolled subjects the trial will have a better chance ('power') of detecting a true benefit.

The high-risk-group approach presents three main problems. First, in order to identify high-risk subjects for a particular cancer, one would need risk factors which are known to be good

predictors of the occurrence of this cancer. A host of risk factors have been identified for most cancers, but few of them, if any, have been shown to be causally involved in the development of these cancers. Speaking of the 'multifactorial aetiology' of cancers is a tribute to our ignorance rather than a proof of our knowledge (Strabanek and McCormick, 1989). For example, countless risk factors have been proposed for breast cancer and the definition of women at high risk of developing breast cancer requires a minimal list of 12 indicators such as prior breast cancer, benign breast disease, breast cancer in a first degree relative, etc. Yet the majority of breast cancers appear in women who do not *a priori* belong to a high-risk group (Henderson, 1990). The second problem lies in the cost of implementing a screening test to locate high-risk subjects. The third problem is the generalizability of the results. Whether benefits seen in high-risk subjects can be transposed to the general population is, in general, debatable (Moon, 1989).

Sample size calculations

The sample size needed in a prevention trial is determined primarily by the magnitude of the effect that can realistically be expected from the intervention. Since the objective of cancer-prevention trials is to reduce the occurrence of rare events, and since the expected benefit of most interventions is small, large or even huge numbers of subjects need to be entered in prevention trials. For instance, the Women's Health Trial was proposed to test whether a low-fat diet can reduce the incidence of breast cancer among high-risk women. It was estimated that over the 10-year duration of the trial, 3.32% of the women in the control group would develop breast cancer (Self *et al.*, 1988). The sample size of 32,000 women was calculated to allow the detection of a reduction in this percentage to 2.77% in the intervention group (i.e. a 0.55% difference between the control and the intervention group).

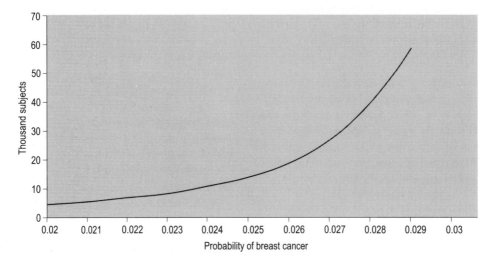

Figure 4   Number of subjects required in a trial of dietary fat reduction for the prevention of breast cancer. Women in the control group are assumed to have a 3.32% probability of developing breast cancer over a 10-year period. The figure shows the number of subjects which would be required to detect various probabilities of developing cancer in the intervention group (assuming a statistical power of 80% at a two-tailed significance level of 5%).

Figure 4 shows that the sample size required is in fact extremely sensitive to the postulated difference between the two groups. For instance, if the target percentage in the intervention group was changed to 2.87% instead of 2.77% (i.e. a reduction of 0.45% instead of 0.55%), more than 50,000 women would be required. Hence a mere 0.1% change in the assumed benefit causes the required sample size to almost double!

Monitoring of prevention trials

Overall monitoring

The monitoring of a prevention trial should include:

1 the monitoring of subject recruitment;

2 the regular assessment of exposure to the intervention (e.g. the regular intake of pills, or the modification of dietary habits);

3 the collection of data on the end-point of interest (cancer incidence, disease-specific mortality or behavioural modification);

4 the collection of data on any expected or unexpected side-effects of the intervention (monitoring after the end of the study is recommended to safeguard against possible long-term consequences of the intervention).

If recruitment does not progress as planned, if compliance is excessively poor, or if the occurrence of end-points is well below the expected rate, measures can be taken or the design of the trial considered (e.g. by increasing the study duration, or by focusing on high-risk subjects). A Data Monitoring Committee is usually asked to advise on early trial termination if a clear benefit or harm is demonstrated before the anticipated end of the trial.

Monitoring of compliance

A careful assessment of exposure to the intervention is critical in explanatory trials aimed at determining a causal relationship between the intervention and the end-point of interest. In these trials the question of interest is: 'Does the intervention work if given as intended?' In pragmatic trials, the actual compliance of the subjects to the intervention is useful in assessing the effectiveness of the intervention. In these trials the question is: 'Can the intervention actually be delivered?'

Compliance to the intervention is seldom a yes/no phenomenon. In dietary trials, for instance, subjects may comply to the intervention to varying degrees, which makes it difficult to quantify their exact exposure to the intervention. Special attention should be paid to drop-ins and drop-outs, as these will dilute any true effect of the intervention. In this respect, the subjects in the control group must receive as much attention as the subjects in the intervention group.

Monitoring of end-points

A trial registry is an essential tool for monitoring the occurrence of end-points among the subjects entered into a prevention trial taking place in the community. The trial registry should permit the linkage between national records on cancer incidence and the subjects in the trial. In countries where no population-based cancer registry exists, a special registry has to be created for the purposes of the trial. The trial registry should also permit the linkage between national death records and the subjects in the trial (the individual date of death is available in most national registries, but the cause of death is not). By the end of the trial, the health status of all subjects entered into the trial should be ascertained, including that of drop-outs. A system to trace individual subjects should be foreseen (e.g. by mail or telephone) even when linkage to national records is possible.

Concluding remarks

It has been estimated that smoking causes about one-third of cancer deaths in western countries, and that dietary factors were implicated in at least another third (Doll and Peto, 1981). Cancer is thus, in theory, a largely preventable disease, Yet, with the exception of

smoking cessation campaigns, no successful prevention programme has thus far been implemented. Two distinct reasons may explain this apparently paradoxical situation. The first is that, in spite of the massive indirect evidence of the role played by dietary factors, few individual factors have been identified unequivocally to be major contributors to the cancer process. The second reason is that, even when there is compelling evidence for a proposed intervention, the reliable confirmation of its benefit through randomized trials is an enormously expensive and lengthy undertaking. This paper has outlined the major difficulties involved in the planning, conduct and interpretation of prevention trials in cancer.

It is fair to say that the background against which prevention trials are proposed today is rather bleak. The only single-factor, randomized trial of anti-smoking advice to current smokers failed to show a statistically significant benefit of the intervention in terms of cardiovascular deaths and lung-cancer deaths (Rose, 1982). The trial had accrued only 1445 subjects, and was thus too small to reach significance, but somewhat encouragingly, it did show a statistically significant increase in deaths due to non-lung cancers among the intervention group! In contrast to the scarcity of cancer prevention trials, there has been a profusion of prevention programmes against cardiovascular disease. These programmes mainly consisted of reductions in cigarette smoking and changes in diet, the major risk factors for cardiovascular disease, and also important causes of cancers. When information on cancer deaths was combined from all available prevention trials in cardiovascular disease, no clear trend emerged either in favour of or against the interventions (Hakama et al., 1990). No randomized trial of a dietary intervention designed primarily to reduce cancer has yet been carried out. The trials that have been proposed have met with considerable resistance because of their monumental cost, even when preliminary trials had shown the feasibility of the intervention (Cullen, 1990). The picture is more encouraging for chemoprevention trials, of which there are two dozen in progress, mostly under the sponsorship of the US National Cancer Institute (Hakama *et al.*, 1990).

Whether or not one believes in the promise that large reductions in cancer deaths can be brought about through prevention programmes, it is essential that the proposed programmes be evaluated in randomized trials. These trials represent major efforts which will only be possible through co-operation on a European, if not a world-wide scale.

References

Alexander, F., Roberts, M.M., Lutz, W. *et al.* (1989) Randomization by cluster and the problem of social calls bias, *J. Epidemiol. and Community Hlth.* **43**, 29–36.

Anzai, Y., Holinka, C.F., Kuramoto, H. and Gurpide, E. (1989) Stimulatory effects of 4-hydroxytamoxifen on proliferation of human endometrial adenocarcinoma cells (Ishikawa line), *Cancer Res.* **49**, 2362–2365.

Boccardo, F., Guarnieri, D., Rubagotti, A., *et al.* (1984) Endocrine effects of tamoxifen in postmenopausal breast cancer patients, *Tumori* **70**, 61–68.

Boyd, N.F., Cousins, M., Lockwood, G. and Tritchler, D. (1990) The feasibility of testing experimentally the dietary fat–breast cancer hypothesis, *Br. J. Cancer* **62**, 878–881.

Buring, H.E. and Hennekens, C.H. (1989) Methodologic issues in the design of primary prevention trials. In *Advances in cancer control: innovations and research.*, Alan R. Liss, New York, 41–49.

Byar, D.P. and Freedman, L.S. (1990) The importance and nature of cancer prevention trials, *Seminars in Oncology* **17**, 413–424.

Cullen, J.W. (1990) Phases in cancer control: intervention research. In Hakama, M. *et al.* (eds.) *Evaluating effectiveness of primary prevention of cancer*. IARC Scientific Publications No. 103, Lyon.

Doll, R. and Peto, R. (1981) *The causes of cancer*, Oxford University Press, Oxford.

Fornander, T., Cedermark, B., Mattson, A. *et al.* (1989) Adjuvant tamoxifen in early breast cancer: occurrence of new primary cancers, *Lancet* **21**, 117–120.

Freedman, L.S. and Green, S.B. (1990) Statistical designs for investigating several interventions in the same study: methods for cancer prevention trials, *J. Nat. Cancer Inst.* **82**, 910–914.

Gottardis, M.M., Robinson, S.P., Satyaswaroop, P.G., Jordan, V.C. (1988) Constrasting actions of tamoxifen on endometrial and breast tumour growth in the athymic mouse, *Cancer Res.* **48**, 812–815.

Greenwald, P., Nixon, D.W., Malone, W.F. *et al.* (1990) Concepts in cancer chemoprevention research, *Cancer* **65**, 1483–1490.

Hakama, M., Beral, V., Cullen, J.W. and Parkin, D.M. (eds.) (1990) *Evaluating effectiveness of primary prevention of cancer*. IARC Scientific Publications No. 103, Lyon.

Hardell, L. (1990) Tamoxifen as a risk factor for endometrial cancer, *Cancer* **65**, 1661.

Henderson, C.I. (1990) What can a women do about her risk of dying of breast cancer, *Curr. Probl. Cancer* July/August, 163–230.

Killacke, M.A., Hakes, T.B. and Pierce, V.K. (1985) Endometrial adenocarcinoma in breast cancer patients receiving antioestrogens, *Cancer Treat. Rep.* **69**, 237–238.

Lopez, A.D. (1990) Changes in tobacco consumption and lung cancer risk: evidence from national statistics. In Hakama, M. *et al.*, (eds.) *Evaluating effectiveness of primary prevention of cancer*. IARC Scientific Publications No. 103, Lyon.

Moon, T.E. (1989) Interpretation of cancer prevention trials, *Preventive Med.* **18**, 721–731.

Nolvadex Adjuvant Trial Organization (1988) Controlled trial of tamoxifen as a single adjuvant agent in the management of early breast cancer, *Br. J. Cancer* **57**, 608–611.

Powles, T.J., Hardy, J.R., Ashley, S.E. *et al.* (1989) A pilot trial to evaluate the acute toxicity and feasibility of tamoxifen for prevention of breast cancer, *Br. J. Cancer* **60**, 126–131.

Prentice, R.L. (1990) Tamoxifen as a potential preventive agent in healthy postmenopausal women, *J. Natl. Cancer Inst.* **82**, 1310–1311.

Ribeiro, G. and Swindell, R. (1988) Christie Hospital adjuvant tamoxifen trial, *Br. J. Cancer* **57**, 601–603.

Rose, G., Hamilton, P.J.S., Cowell, L. and Shipley, M.J. (1982) A randomized controlled trial of anti-smoking advice: 10-year results, *J. Epidemiol. Com. Hlth.* **36**, 102–108.

Self, S., Prentice, R., Iverson, D. *et al.* (1988) Statistical design of the Women's Health Trial, *Controlled Clin. Trials* **9**, 119–136.

Smith, D.C., Prentice, R., Thompson, D.J. and Herrman, W.L. (1975) Association of exogenous estrogen and endometrial carcinoma, *N. Engl. J. Med.* **293**, 1164–1167.

Steering Committee of the Physicians' Health Study Research Group (1988) Preliminary report: findings from the Aspirin component of the ongoing physicians' health study, *N. Engl. J. Med.* **318**, 262–264.

Strabanek, P., McCormick, J. (1989) *Follies and fallacies in medicine*, The Tarragon Press, Glasgow.

Trock, B., Lanza, E. and Greenwald, P. (1990) Dietary fibre, vegetables and colon cancer: critical review and meta-analyses of the epidemiological evidence, *J. Natl. Cancer Inst.* **82**, 650–661.

Willett, W.C., Stampfer, M.J., Colditz, G.A. *et al.* (1990) Relation of meat, fat and fibre intake to the risk of colon cancer in a prospective study among women, *N. Engl. J. Med.* **323**, 1664–1672.

Zelen, M. (1988) Are primary cancer prevention trials feasible? *J. Natl. Cancer Inst.* **80**, 1442–1444.

Ziehl, H. and Finkle, W.D. (1975) Increased risk of endometrial carcinoma among users of conjugated estrogens, *N. Engl. J. Med.* **293**, 1164–1167.

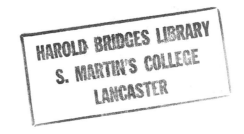
HAROLD BRIDGES LIBRARY
S. MARTIN'S COLLEGE
LANCASTER

1 . 4

RELIABILITY OF CANCER DATA

Calum Muir

Introduction

Two main sources of information about cancer are mortality, i.e. the number of deaths ascribed to the disease, and incidence, the number of newly diagnosed cases occurring in a defined population. Each of these complementary sources has its advantages and drawbacks. Mortality data have existed in most western European countries since the turn of the century. Incidence data were rarely available before 1940, and for the majority of countries not until around 1960.

Mortality is influenced by the efficacy of treatment but is usually complete, in that people die but once and the cause of death is usually recorded. Figures of incidence depend on the effectiveness of the registration system and coverage tends to be patchy. National registries exist in the United Kingdom and Denmark, for example, while in France, Spain and Italy only a comparatively small proportion of the population is covered. In this paper, we assess the reliability of these two principal sources of cancer data and list the questions that should be asked when using these sources of information.

Mortality data

The fact of death is formally recorded in all EC countries and Death Certificates are accompanied by or include the opinion of a medically qualified person on the underlying cause of death. It is this opinion which is coded by the current revision of the International Classification of Disease (WHO, 1978) and eventually tabulated to create lists of causes of death by disease, age and sex. Errors can be introduced at many levels.

The cause of death given by the certifying physician may not be correct. There have been many studies in which persons who would normally sign a Death Certificate were asked to do so on a dummy certificate before a postmortem was carried out. The results of the postmortem were then compared with what would have been on the certificate if the postmortem had not taken place. Not only were cancers not diagnosed when they existed, but they were also considered to be present when they were not. Not infrequently, the site of cancer given was incorrect. Inaccuracies tended to increase with advancing age (Cameron and McGoogan, 1981). This and other studies (Heasman and Lipworth, 1946; Goldman et al., 1983) have shown that although the diagnosis may be incorrect for a proportion of individuals, when over-registrations and under-registrations are taken into account, the totals are remarkably little changed. While the statistical picture may be on balance correct, for epidemiological studies in which groups of exposed individuals are followed to ascertain their cause of death, the fate of the individual becomes more important.

In some cultures, there may still be a reluctance to write the word 'cancer' on a Death Certificate and the extent of this can only be assessed by ad hoc study. The existence of such reluctance may be suspected when the proportion of cancer deaths which do not give a statement on the organ affected is high. Such deaths are typically ascribed to 'cancer' or 'malignant neoplasm'. In tabulations these deaths appear under the ICD rubrics 195–199.

Sometimes Death Certificates are difficult to interpret in that the certifier may not be clear. This may result in the Death Certificate coder having to reach an arbitrary decision as to what was meant. In several countries, such as the UK, however, it is possible to query vague and doubtful diagnoses. Provision may be made on the Death Certificate to indicate that a postmortem will be held and that more complete information will be available after completion of the autopsy. In general, where such follow-back schemes exist, the quality of death certification is better. In European countries (for example, in France) where the medically certified cause of death is separated from the identify of the deceased such follow-back schemes are impossible.

In an illuminating study, Percy et al. (1981) examined the Death Certificates of persons known to have cancer and whose Certificates mentioned this fact. Despite the precise information available from the cancer registration system, this was not always carried over to the Death Certificate. Cancer of the rectum (ICD8 154) became cancer of the large bowel (and hence coded to ICD8 153) and specified leukaemia became leukaemia NOS.

International comparison of cancer data may be strongly influenced by national differences in coding practice. Taking a set of 1,234 US Death Certificates mentioning cancer as the cause of death, national Vital Statistics Offices in nine countries – USA, Canada, England and Wales, Brazil, France, Federal Republic of Germany, Netherlands, USSR and New Zealand – were asked to code the same certificates. There were quite surprising differences, even for cancers such as those of the breast, due largely to differences in interpretation of the meaning of 'underlying cause of death' (Percy and Muir, 1989).

In the past five years, the European Community has been studying the effect of inaccuracies of death certification and coding practices on observed differences in international mortality statistics. A recent study of cancer (Kelson and Farebrother, 1987) incorporated a further step compared with most other accuracy of cause of death studies in that physicians were asked to complete Death Certificates from the same case histories which were then coded by National Offices of Vital Statistics and the World Health

Organization reference centre. This showed that doctors did not necessarily fill out the Death Certificates similarly from the same case history – introducing yet another discrepancy to be taken into consideration in comparing mortality statistics. Perhaps the most serious problem to emerge was the failure to distinguish between cancer of the cervix and cancer of the uterus, a problem reported over 20 years ago.

These factors can have considerable differences on international comparisons. The problem is complex and multi-faceted. A major obstacle is unthinking certification of death, rather than lack of knowledge of diagnosis, the value of the Death Certificate for many purposes being unrecognized. The coders must rely on what is written on the Death Certificate.

The person scrutinizing mortality data should ask the following questions: Is death registration complete? Is the cause of death for all deceased persons given by medical practitioners? If so, is there a follow-back system for incorporating further information following autopsy or query by the Vital Statistics Office? Attention should be given to the proportion of all deaths from vague and ill-certificated causes (as such deaths may include persons with cancer) and to the proportion of cancer deaths for which site of origin is not given (as this may reflect lack of precision in diagnosis or careless certification). To quote Smithers (1960): 'Cancer mortality statistics must be seen for what they are, which is a summary of what thousands of doctors of varying skill have, under very different conditions and opportunities for accurate diagnosis, seen fit to write as their opinion of the cause of death.'

The age-specific mortality rates for the commoner sites would normally rise smoothly with age. The failure of the age-specific mortality rates to rise in this manner may reflect under-diagnosis of cancer in older people or the existence of a birth cohort effect, people dying at older ages not having been exposed to the same quantity of carcinogenic agents as younger persons.

Incidence data

Information on the incidence of cancer is relatively sparse compared to that for mortality and further covers much shorter periods of time. National coverage is the exception rather than the rule, and is available only for the Nordic countries, Great Britain, Canada, the former German Democratic Republic, Australia, New Zealand and Singapore. In Poland and the USSR, there is national registration but it is recognized that the quality is uneven.

While registries endeavour to ensure that all cases of cancer are reported to them, in practice this is probably never realized. Most registries, however, would hope to cover around 95% of cases. While there have been several ingenious mathematical methods to assess the extent of under-registration, these are probably no better than the classical indicators of precision of diagnosis and of completeness of registration which are:

(a) the proportion of notifications with age unknown, – which should normally be very low (age may be missing on notifications for non-melanoma skin cancer, which is frequently diagnosed on an outpatient basis) (see below);

(b) the proportion of diagnoses with histological verification (frequently denoted as HV per cent in publications) implies that a portion of the tumour has been removed and after processing cut into very thin slices which are stained by a variety of dyes. The resulting section is then examined under the microscope by a histopathologist. While ideally all suspected tumours should be so examined, other reliable methods of diagnosis exist, for example radiology for cancer of the oesophagus, biochemical measurements such as serum foetoprotein levels for primary liver cancer, etc. A very high proportion of histologically verified

cases may either indicate that all suspected cases of cancer are thoroughly investigated or reflect the fact that the registry is only receiving notifications from pathologists and is not covering adequately cancer patients diagnosed by other means. The definition of histological verification may vary between registries. Some would include only microscopic examination of tissue removed from the tumour. Others extend the definition to smears made from bone marrow, from blood or from fluid, for example in the pleural and abdominal cavities. Smears taken from the cervix uteri are not usually considered as histological verification even though these may be reported as 'positive'. When comparing registries, the definitions used for HV should be checked (see Muir *et al.*, 1987).

(c) DCO (Death Certificate Only) per cent denotes the proportion of all notifications for which the only information available to the cancer registry is a statement on a Death Certificate that a deceased person has cancer. This is usually less than 5% in most registries. A raised frequency of DCO registrations not only shows that the registry may be missing cases, but can also indicate where losses are taking place and where remedial action should be directed. Unfortunately, this most useful index of data quality is not available in those countries in which privacy legislation prohibits the use of Death Certificates in cancer registration. The inability to make the link between Death Certificates and registered cases of cancer also means that it is not possible to calculate the survival for a population using conventional methods (see also below).

(d) the relationship between mortality and incidence for a given cancer in the registration area at a particular time (M/I per cent). This varies considerably from site to site, being close to unity for rapidly fatal forms of malignancy, such as those of the oesophagus, and very low for non-melanoma skin cancers. If mortality and incidence are close for cancers known to have good survival, under-registration should be suspected.

Many of these indicators are age-dependent. Histological verification is normally very high and DCO percentage very low in younger persons: typical values are given in Figure 1. Even in the records of the SEER (Surveillance, Epidemiology and End Results) registries of the US, a resource co-ordinated by the US National Cancer Institute, after 75 years of age there is a gradual diminution in the proportion on clinical grounds alone and in the proportion registered on the basis of a Death Certificate only (Muir, 1990).

Diagnosis and notification of cancers

For a case of cancer to be registered, the disease must be diagnosed. This implies both a willingness of the person concerned to seek medical advice and the availability and ability of a health-care system to make the diagnosis. In some cultures, there is a degree of reluctance, notably among older persons and possibly to a greater extent among women, to seek medical advice, believing that their symptoms are a natural concomitant of advancing age. Among the medical profession there may be a greater reluctance to investigate and treat the elderly, either because resources are scarce or there is no

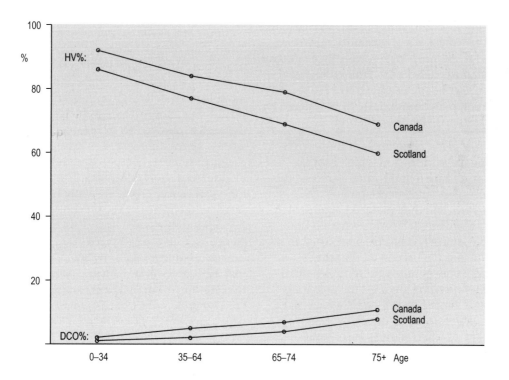

Figure 1 Indicators of reliability of cancer incidence data around 1980 by broad age group, males, Scotland and Canada.
HV%: proportion of incident cases with histological confirmation of diagnosis.
DCO%: proportion of incident cases for which the only evidence available to the cancer registry was a statement on a death certificate that the deceased had cancer.

wish to submit the elderly to invasive and on occasion, uncomfortable procedures to make a diagnosis, an attitude which would normally be reflected in the HV per cent index. For an increasing number of cancer sites, diagnosis and treatment are carried out on an outpatient basis, the most frequent of these being non-melanoma skin cancer. For this reason, many registries do not seek information on this form of malignancy which, although of low fatality, consumes sizeable amounts of medical care. Unless special efforts are made, it is possible to lose cancers dealt with solely at outpatients clinics. Frequently, the first indication of the existence of such cases is a pathology report.

Once the diagnosis of cancer is made, this fact has to be reported to the registry. The mechanisms for doing so vary substantially. The physician making the diagnosis fills in a notification form transmitting this in confidence to the registry. Such responsibility may be devolved to the hospital records office or some other administrative body. Trained registry staff may visit hospitals to extract case records. Registration may be voluntary or mandated by administrative order or legislation.

However, it is the motivation of those supplying the information which is of greatest significance. Once a notification is received by a cancer registry and checked for completeness, it is then matched against existing records to determine whether the individual concerned has been reported to the registry before. To make sure that the individual is not counted twice, a variety of items of information are used for matching records, the most valuable of which are name, date of birth, place of birth, sex or unique identifying numbers such as exist in the Nordic countries.

The items used for such matches are often dictated by local legislation and customs. It may be possible to match, as in Scotland, all hospital discharge diagnoses with the more detailed notifications sent to the cancer registries. The data analyst should thus have a knowledge of the practice at the registries he is

interested in to assess whether any differences in incidence observed could be due to registration procedure.

A wide range of this type of information is tabulated in the Cancer Incidence in Five Continents monographs (Muir *et al.*, 1987). Some registries include, for example, benign papilloma of bladder, benign salivary gland tumours and the benign and unspecified brain tumours with the malignant tumours. While such inclusions may not alter the incidence rates substantially, they should nonetheless be known to the data user.

When scrutinizing tables, as for mortality, one looks for a smooth rise with advancing age in the incidence of most cancer. Given the relatively uniform incidence globally, childhood malignancy should fall within the incidence ranges observed in succeeding volumes of Cancer Incidence in Five Continents. Kidney and eye cancer age-incidence curves should reflect the childhood peaks due to nephroblastoma and retinoblastoma. Brain tumours and leukaemia would also show an increase in children, a fall thereafter followed by a sustained rise in adults. Normally there would be a two-fold excess of females compared with males for gall bladder and thyroid cancers. The incidence rate for colon cancer would be equal in the two sexes, while rectum cancer usually shows a two-fold male excess. Uterus NOS should comprise a very small proportion of uterine cancer. Very low levels of, say, brain cancer may reflect no more than an absence of the relevant means of diagnosis and a sudden increase may reflect the arrival of a neurosurgeon.

It is worth remembering that during the first two years or so of a registry's existence there may be under-reporting as the system is being set up. There may also be over-reporting of persons with cancer diagnosed in earlier years being erroneously considered to be incident cases. Once the registry is established, one would not expect to see major year-to-year fluctuations in incidence for the major sites.

Systematic scrutiny of age-specific incidence rates is worth while as changes in either direction are often first seen in the younger age group, as it is the young who first take up a new habit or give up an established one, for example smoking (Muir *et al.*, 1981; Doll, 1988). Unfortunately, it is in these age groups that statistical fluctuations are most likely, a problem which can be minimized by the use of the rolling three-year average or statistical modelling. A well run registry would make periodical checks to ensure that the pattern of reporting by source had not changed significantly.

There is no universally applicable set of rules to assess registry data. If in doubt, data users should consult the registry in question, which is likely to know where problems may lie.

While statistical data on cancer have many potential sources of error and bias, they are undoubtedly much more reliable than for any other category of disease. In many countries, around 90% of cancer diagnoses are confirmed by histological examination of a portion of disease taken from the tumours. While mortality data are less accurate, they are nonetheless available for long periods of time. Taken together, these two sources give an excellent picture of the disease which is responsible for one in four deaths in much of the world.

References

Cameron, H.W. and McGoogan, C. (1981) Prospective study of 1152 hospital autopsies. Inaccuracies in death certification, *J. Pathol.* **133**, 273–283.

Doll, R. (1988) Epidemiology and the prevention of cancer: some recent developments, *J. Cancer Res. Clin. Oncol.* **116**, 447–458.

Fujimoto, I. and Hanai, A. (1987) Comparability and quality of data: reliability of registration. In Muir *et al.* (1987) loc. cit., 45–59.

Goldman, L., Sayson, R., Robbins, S., Cohn, L.H., Bothmann, M. and Weisberg, M. (1983) Value of autopsy in three medical eras, *New Eng. J. Med.* **308**, 1000–1005.

Heasman, M.A and Lipworth, L. (1946) Accuracy of certification of cause of death. Studies on medical and population subjects No. 20, HMSO, London.

Kelson, M. and Farebrother, M. (1987) The effect of inaccuracies in death certification and coding practices in the European Economic Community (EEC) on international cancer mortality statistics, *Int. J. Epidemiol.* **16**, 411–414.

Muir, C. (1990) Geographical patterns of cancer: role of environment. In Macieira-Coelho, A. and Nordenskjöld, B. (eds.) (1990) *Cancer and ageing*, CRC Press, Boca Raton.

Muir, C., Waterhouse, J., Mack, T., Powell, J. and Whelan, S. (1987) *Cancer incidence in five continents, Volume V*. IARC Scientific Publication No. 88, International Agency for Research on Cancer, Lyon.

Muir, C.S., Choi, N.W. and Schifflers, G. (1981) Time trends in cancer mortality in some countries and their possible causes and significance. In *Proceedings of Skandia International Symposium*, Almqvist and Wiksell Int., Stockholm, Sweden, 269–309.

Percy, C. and Muir, C.S. (1989) The international comparability of cancer mortality data and results of an international death certificate study, *Am. J. Epidemiol.* **129**, 936–944.

Percy, C., Stanek, C. and Gloeckler, L. (1981) Accuracy of cancer death certificates and the effect on cancer mortality statistics, *Am. J. Publ. Hlth.* **71**, 242–250.

Smithers, D.W. (1960) *Monographs on neoplastic disease – introductory volume. A clinical prospect of the cancer problem*, Edinburgh, Livingstone.

A SIMPLIFIED BIOLOGY OF CANCERS

Malcolm Taylor

Introduction

In some of our normal body tissues, such as bone marrow and the small bowel, cells are turning over quite rapidly, that is that they are dying and being replaced by new cells. These normal cells show a tightly controlled regulation of growth. In contrast, cancer cells show uncontrolled growth. This need not be fast growth, but it is relentless and has two further important characteristics; firstly, an ability to invade and destroy adjacent normal tissue, and secondly, an ability to seed to sites in the body distant from the original tumour. It is this invasion and metastasis (seeding) of a tumour that is the most life-threatening aspect of cancer formation or oncogenesis.

Cancer can occur in any tissue of the body. This means there are many different types of cancer, each quite different in character from the others; some are slower growing, some faster, some are more destructive or quicker to metastasize; some are more amenable to treatment than others. Even within a single tissue, different types of cancer can be distinguished, for example different forms of leukaemia can arise from bone marrow cells, depending on their cell type and stage of maturation.

Cancer is not inherited. In some rare families, however, there may be a greatly increased likelihood for certain individuals to develop a particular form of cancer as a result of the genes he or she has inherited, for example in some families with a high incidence of breast cancer.

If cancer arises as a result of the loss of cellular control of growth, we might ask what causes this. It is now generally agreed that cancer cells arise following a sequence of separate abnormal genetic changes (mutations) in the DNA. Several such changes spread over many years are required to be expressed in a single cell for it to become cancerous, which explains why, with some exceptions, cancer incidence increases with age. Because changes are necessary in the genetic material, we can say that at the cellular level cancer is a genetic disease. Let us consider the broad evidence that cancer is a genetic disorder in this sense.

If a series of say three, four, five or six genetic changes is required in a single cell and they all have to be accumulated before a tumour can be initiated, then we might expect that if the final mutation does not occur, the tumour will not develop. We can consider, for example, cigarette smoking to contribute in some unknown way to these genetic changes in lung cells which culminate in lung cancer. Over many years, different cells in the lungs undergo genetic damage with continued smoking until eventually one cell accumulates all the necessary mutations and is able to trigger a cancerous growth. If a smoker gives up the habit, even after many years of smoking, he or she will have a reduced risk of developing lung cancer compared with the risk from continued smoking. The inference is that there is a late step necessary for tumour formation which is avoided by this action. This effect can only be detected by looking at large populations of people but nevertheless this epidemiological evidence is consistent with the notion that cancer requires several distinct genetic steps for its development.

More direct evidence comes from observations on tumour cells. Chromosomes carry the genetic material of the cell and are responsible for transmitting DNA from parent cell from one generation to the next in the eggs and sperm. Many tumours, particularly leukaemias, are characterized by very consistent chromosomal abnormalities. For example, in chronic myeloid leukaemia (CML) there is a consistent reciprocal exchange or translocation of genetic material between chromosomes 9 and 22 in almost all cases of this tumour (Figure 1). The very close association of this specific genetic alteration with a particular tumour type suggests that this genetic change is important in the development of the tumour. There are many other similar examples.

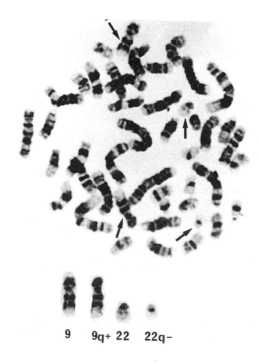

9   9q+ 22   22q−

Figure 1   Human chromosome spread from a patient with chronic myeloid leukaemia, indicating the translocation chromosomes

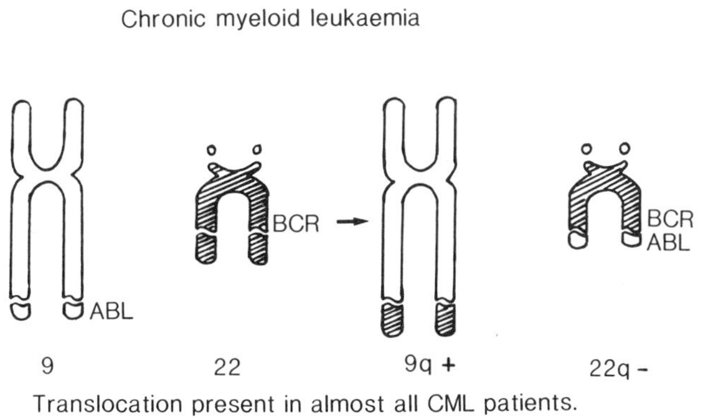

Chronic myeloid leukaemia

9   22   9q +   22q −

Translocation present in almost all CML patients.

Figure 2   Diagram of the exchange between chromosomes 9 and 22 in CML

Table 1 Some proto-oncogenes associated with human tumours

Proto-oncogene	Tumour	Mechanism of activation
ABL	Chronic myeloid leukaemia	Chromosome translocation
NEU	Adenocarcinoma of breast	Gene amplification
MYC	Burkitts lymphoma	Chromosome translocation
L-MYC	Carcinoma of lung	Gene amplification
N-MYC	Neuroblastoma	Gene amplification
H-RAS	Colon cancer	Point mutation
K-RAS	Acute myeloid leukaemia	Point mutation

Thirdly, if any single tumour is examined, it can usually be shown that all the tumour cells are genetically identical or form a clone. This observation is consistent with the idea that one cell originally underwent some crucial genetic change which gave it the properties we associate with a cancerous cell, and then grew into the tumour we recognize. Tumours do not seem to arise from many cells that simultaneously go through the oncogenic process.

From these different lines of evidence, therefore, we can be certain that cancer does involve a series of changes in the DNA of individual cells.

Mechanisms by which genetic change may lead to cancerous cells

There are many mechanisms by which such genetic change occurs, which is not surprising bearing in mind the many different types of cell, all with different normal functions, that can become cancerous. The involvement of a chromosome exchange in the development of chronic myeloid leukaemia was mentioned above. In order to appreciate the importance of this exchange we have to turn from the level of the whole chromosome to the molecular level. As a result of the break in chromosome 9, a gene called ABL is brought into a new

juxtaposition with another genetic region (Figure 2) (BCR on chromosome 22).

An entirely new gene is formed in the process by the fusion of hitherto separated regions. As a result, a new protein is produced, which is not found in normal cells, and in some way contributes to the leukaemogenic process. ABL is termed a cellular proto-oncogene. Although the precise function of this gene in its normal location is unknown, it plays an important role in development because it is found in many different organisms showing it has been conserved during evolution. Over sixty different proto-oncogenes have now been described (see Table 1).

Different proto-oncogenes have a normal role in different cell types and in different stages of differentiation. ABL is one of the many cellular proto-oncogenes which appears to have a role in oncogenesis if conditions allow. The chromosome translocation in CML is said to activate the proto-oncogene to abnormal gene expression.

All proto-oncogenes have an important general feature in common they are involved in some way in normal cell growth or differentiation. Genetic alteration of the proto-oncogene is likely, therefore, to profoundly affect the growth responses of the cell. Regulated normal cell growth is a remarkably complex process involving the interaction between factors external to the cell (growth factors, differentiation factors, hormones, etc.) and the cell's response to them. Growth factors require receptors on the target cell surface in order to bring about a response in the cell. For a growth factor to affect gene expression in the cell, a message must be transmitted from the cell membrane across the cytoplasm and into the nucleus (Figure 3). All these intricate processes are mediated by the products of different proto-oncogenes.

An important feature of activated proto-oncogenes is that they show their effect when only one of the two alleles is mutated, i.e. they

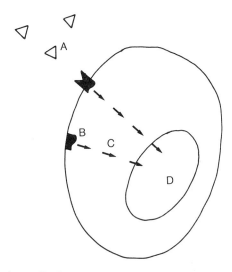

Figure 3 Site of action in the cell of oncogene products. A, as growth factors; B, as part of a growth factor receptor of the cell membrane; C, as part of the signal transducing process across the cytoplasm; D, as a nuclear factor

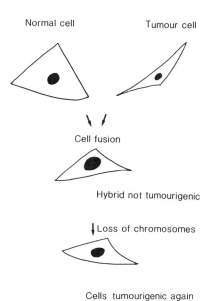

Figure 4 Diagram illustrating cell fusion

act in a dominant fashion. Of course, one oncogene acting in an appropriate way represents only one abnormal genetic change, and additional changes are required to produce the cancer cell. Some activated oncogenes may have their effect early in initiating malignant change, while others act later in the sequence of events. Amplification of the number of copies of some proto-oncogenes appears to be an important later step in oncogenesis.

Suppressor genes

There is a second type of cancer gene which can be contrasted with proto-oncogenes. These genes function to suppress the oncogenic tendency of other genes and are therefore termed **suppressor genes**. Early studies showed that when malignant cells were fused with normal cells in tissue culture, the resulting hybrid cells were not tumorigenic (Figure 4). No gene has so far been identified that is responsible for the suppression of tumour growth by cell fusion. The occurrence of suppression has been taken as evidence that cancer cells contain recessive genes involved in tumorigenesis. A second important finding concerning the existence of suppressor genes came from studies of an embryonic tumour, of immature retinocytes in the eye, called retinoblastoma. Interestingly, there is a genetic predisposition to retinoblastoma which is inherited as an autosomal dominant trait and is seen in about 40% of all retinoblastoma cases. It was proposed that in this inherited or familial form of retinoblastoma the affected individual inherited a mutant allele (with loss of function) from the affected parent and this allele therefore is present in every cell in the body. Subsequently, a spontaneous (somatic) mutation occurred that inactivated the second allele derived from the normal parent. The frequency of spontaneous mutations is high enough that almost all patients inheriting the predisposition develop at least one tumour.

In the sporadic or non-familial form of the tumour, it was proposed that two spontaneous mutational events, one in each allele, must occur in a single retinocyte. This combination is less likely, and generally only single tumours occur. In retinoblastoma, therefore, both alleles at a particular suppressor gene locus undergo mutation, leading to total loss of function at that locus and allowing a tumour to develop (Figure 5). This hypothesis has been substantiated experimentally using both cytogenic and molecular techniques. Separate genetic events are indeed responsible for inactivating each of the two alleles within a tumour.

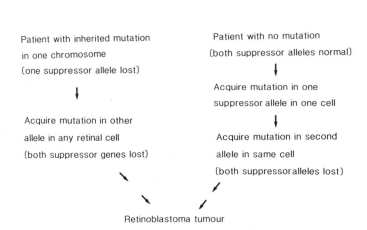

Figure 5 Genetic steps involved in the development of retinoblastoma

A third important piece of evidence supporting the idea of tumour suppressor genes arose from the work on retinoblastoma. Analysis of chromosomes, enzymatic markers and DNA markers in a range of more common tumours (including breast and lung cancer) showed that these tumours had lost part or all of a chromosome. For any single tumour type the loss involved the same chromosome. The inference of this observation was that this represented loss of the normal suppressor gene allele, leaving the other allele which was in some way already inactivated and non-functional. This process is termed loss of heterozygosity, since the tumour cell is effectively homozygous for a particular gene (termed hemizygous if only one chromosome is present). Analysing loss of heterozygosity is important because it has been used to indicate the chromosomal location of suppressor genes predisposing to different tumours.

There is a growing number of suppressor genes implicated in oncogenesis in man (see Table 2). One further example of a very common tumour involving suppressor gene loss is colonic cancer. In both the familial form of this tumour (familial adenomatosis polyposis – FAP) and the non-familial form, loss of several different suppressor genes has been described. In this disorder there is progression to a malignant phenotype via an initially benign proliferation. The mode of action of suppressor genes can be quite complex.

Table 2 Some suppressor genes associated with human tumours

Suppressor gene	Tumour
RB1	Retinoblastoma
	Osteosarcoma
p53	Carcinoma of breast, lung
WT1	Wilms tumour (embryonic kidney tumour)
DCC	Carcinoma of colon
FA1	Carcinoma of colon

The precise biochemical mechanisms by which any suppressor gene product regulates cell behaviour is not known in detail. Some gene products may regulate passage of the cell through the cell cycle. (The RB gene product may regulate entry of cells into DNA synthesis). Other suppressor gene products may be DNA-binding proteins with roles in regulating transcription or replication. A third type of product may function in inter-cell interactions.

It is clear that genetic changes in both proto-oncogenes and suppressor genes are important in the development of cancer. Many apparently sequential changes are observed in human tumour cells, and the occurrence of only two such changes is likely to be unusual. In the example of FAP, both oncogene activation and the involvement of three different suppressor genes have so far been implicated.

Why loss of several suppressor genes is required is not understood, but it may be that their products regulate different events. What is the molecular genetics of tumour progression? In the multistep process of tumour development, each genetic event may confer an additional phenotypic abnormality; an enhanced ability for benign proliferation, invasion or metastasis, for example. The processes which drive progression are not well understood. In the case of several tumours, it is possible that they arise as a result of a selection driven process, with some additional increment of phenotypic change observable at each stage (as in FAP). Equally, however, it is possible that the tumour may arise following the accumulation of a particular number of genetic mutations (as, for example, in retinoblastoma). There may be no required order to the acquisition of such changes. Progression does appear to result in loss of some genes and duplication of others. There is an increased likelihood of amplification of some genes, which in turn often heralds a more aggressive form of the disease. It is one of the aims of cancer genetics to link the steps in the pathogenesis of tumour progression to specific genetic lesions.

Interaction of genes with environmental agents to initiate, promote or maintain the genetic change

The common feature of all the cellular changes is genetic change or mutation. How does this occur? Is it a spontaneous process or do interactions with environmental agents produce these mutations? It is known that many chemical carcinogens produce cancer, for example cigarette smoking, vinyl chloride monomer, asbestos, Aflatoxin B, etc. These agents may cause the initiating mutation in the sequence of events leading to cancer development. Physical agents such as X-rays and ultraviolet light are both known to be carcinogens and are known to be able to cause mutation. There is now good evidence that viruses are important in the development of some human cancers, for example human T cell leukaemia virus in adult T cell leukaemia, chronic infection with Hepatitis B virus in liver cancer, Papilloma viruses and Epstein Barr virus. All these agents provide different means of causing the genetic mutation important in cancer development.

Oncogenesis by mutated RAS genes following exposure to chemical carcinogens has been described in experimental systems. There are examples, however, of interactions between environmental agents and specific human genes in producing cancer. One such example is the disorder xeroderma pigmentosum in which patients have an enzyme defect which prevents repair of sunlight (UV) induced damage to their DNA. As a consequence, these patients develop hundreds of cancers only on parts of their bodies exposed to the sun. None of the mutagens described above has been linked directly to the genetic damage found in specific human tumours. In addition to these changes, there are also hormonal influences and immune responses which are important in the progression of tumours.

The use of molecular genetics in clinical practice

Can the information discussed above be put to use in helping to form a diagnosis, a prognosis or providing treatment for cancer patients? In terms of the diagnosis, some chromosome translocations and rearrangements of genes affected by these translocations can be used to help diagnosis of different leukaemias and lymphomas.

Prognostic features have been observed in some tumours, for example amplification and over-expression of the N-MYC oncogene in neuroblastoma is associated with a poorer prognosis. Amplification of the oncogene NEU in breast cancer, however, may not be such a clear indication of prognosis. Secondary chromosome changes in some leukaemias (e.g. CML) are associated with a poor prognosis. Monitoring the patient in this way can, to some degree, supplement the clinical findings.

In terms of treatment, there seems little prospect that repairing damaged oncogenes in cells or replacing deleted suppressor genes will be possible. It is more likely, however, that drugs or some form of immunotherapy may be devised to inhibit activated oncogene proteins. This sort of therapy will probably have to be thought of as a supplement to conventional surgery, chemotherapy, radiotherapy and bone marrow transplantation, etc., in order, for example, to eliminate residual tumour cells.

Looking into the future

Amongst the improved treatments for cancer being tested are genetically engineered haematopoietic growth factors, the use of which may permit increases in the dosages of cytotoxic drugs by lessening bone marrow depression. Continued research will improve our understanding of how genes are involved in cancer development, and at present a great deal of effort is being put into this internationally. Treatment of patients who already have cancer may be different in terms of the prospects for gene therapy, but considerable work is in hand in developing safe animal models.

Gene therapy in the longer term may help the growing number of those known to be at an increased risk of developing a particular cancer. Often these inherited disorders have other severe clinical features. It may be

possible that some gene therapy aimed at ameliorating these other effects will also give these patients some protection against cancer. To leave the situation to the point where cancer develops is too late. In those families where an increased cancer risk is the only clinical feature, gene therapy may again offer more long-term hope.

PART 2

PREVENTABLE CANCERS: SOME CASE STUDIES

INTRODUCTION

The papers in this section examine different types of cancers and a variety of potentially carcinogenic hazards. These are critically examined and the implications for cancer prevention are explored. The subject areas have been chosen to reflect the areas where there is current debate and public discussion, and where there is intensive research activity.

A variety of researchers have estimated that between 30 to 40 percent of all cancers are probably related to nutritional factors. Although the best evidence for this comes from cancers of the colon, rectum and stomach, nutritional factors are thought to be important in the genesis and development of many other cancers. Michael Hill in 'Nutrition and prevention of human cancer' reviews the evidence for this relationship, and discusses research into the possible mechanisms by which nutritional factors could cause human cancers. He discusses the emerging understanding in this area and discusses why it is difficult to undertake effective research. The controversial role of trace elements and vitamins is discussed, as well as the role of food preservatives and additives. Hill concludes that it can be difficult to give authoritative advice on diet to the general public relating specifically to cancers because of the lack of firm evidence in this field. However, it does seem to be emerging that the sort of diet that probably helps to protect individuals from some common cancers is broadly similar to the diet that is important for the prevention of coronary heart disease and other major chronic diseases. There may, therefore, be good grounds for giving general dietary advice and attempting to promote policies favouring healthy food options which will be applicable to many avoidable diseases.

While the incidence of many cancers, for example cancer of the stomach, has been declining throughout Europe, the rise in incidence of malignant melanoma has continued in most of the developed countries of the northern hemisphere. In 'Malignant melanoma – the story unfolds', Rona MacKie charts this rise. She attributes it principally to increased exposure of fair skin to sunlight. This has been brought about by social fashion and patterns of leisure activities, particularly holidaying in very hot countries. A variety of primary and secondary measures for prevention are discussed. Providing more information to the public, providing more shade near places where people relax in the sun, and shielding the skin with appropriate clothing, as well as the vigorous promotion of UV blockers would all help prevent this type of cancer. Early detection and prompt, effective treatment is also important in helping to control the epidemic. Individual people and health professionals, particularly in primary care, should be aware of the presenting features of early malignant melanoma, and understand the necessity for prompt action.

The role of occupational factors in cancer causation has been apparent since Pott described the occurrence of skin cancers in the chimney sweeps of eighteenth century England (Pott, 1775). In 'Occupational cancer prevention', Harri Vainio brings all the work on known occupational carcinogens and their effects up to date. He argues that additional research should continue to determine cancer risk factors at work. This information would bring about the modification of industrial practices for the sake of workers' health. Vainio is aware that such modification raises sensitive issues of regulatory policy, economic welfare and personal freedom. However, he believes that this is worth pursuing as most occupationally related cancers can be prevented by relatively simple means through alterations in work practices and manufacturing processes.

Popular concerns about cancers

Smoking and diet are areas of popular concern about cancers which attract much anxiety and attention. However, there are other kinds of cancer causation which elicit popular concern. In his examination of the dangers posed by low level radiation, Roger Milne looks at some of the sources of radiation to which human beings are exposed. Much exposure comes from natural sources, for example sunlight and radon gas, but artificially created sources, such as medical x-rays, nuclear weapons fall-out, occupational exposure as well as discharge from nuclear installations, also contribute to the total radiation exposure and attract enormous public attention. Cancers caused by radiation probably form a very small proportion of the total number of cancers in most populations. However, it is clear that radiation is a causal factor in some cancers, and it is not clear what a 'safe' dosage of radioactivity might be or the exact mechanism by which it causes those cancers. In the absence of more certain knowledge in this field, Milne argues that it makes sense to minimise exposure to all types of radiation whenever this is possible.

A similar lack of certainty pervades the field of psychological stress and cancers. While many members of the general public may strongly believe that stress and stressful events are crucial in cancer causation, research has so far been unable to establish definite causal connections. Stephen Greer, in 'Stress and psychological aspects of cancers', reviews the evidence of the links between stress and cancer causation. The evidence so far seems to reject the notion that psychological factors directly cause cancers. There is some evidence to suggest that certain kinds of personality

may predispose to cancers, but Greer calls for more research on this issue. Lack of convincing evidence seems to imply that few recommendations can be made for cancer prevention in this area with our current state of knowledge.

Klim McPherson, in 'Hormones and cancers', looks at the evidence for hormonal causative factors in cancers. With the widespread use of exogenous hormones for a variety of therapeutic uses, for example for control of symptoms during the menopause and for contraception, it is important to determine if there are any links between their usage and cancer production. Evidence is slowly emerging, and this is reviewed by McPherson. Quite complex patterns seem to exist and, although some hormones do appear to increase the risk of certain cancers, they may at the same time be protective for other types of cancers. The same hormones that appear to increase the risk of some cancers may also be protective for other types of potentially serious disease, for example coronary heart disease and osteoporosis. Just looking at cancers is not sufficient when trying to determine overall risk factors for individual people. The research required to establish precise risk patterns requires many years of strenuous effort following large numbers of people undertaking a variety of different interventions.

Tobacco and cancers

Although the dangers of tobacco consumption in cancer causation are now increasingly well-known, no book on prevention in this area would be complete without paying some attention to this subject.

The tobacco-related pandemic is of grave concern to all those involved in health promotion. One third of cancers are directly caused by smoking and other kinds of tobacco consumption. The nature of the threat posed from this direction is explored in the paper 'Tobacco and cancers', an edited version of a pamphlet written by international experts from the World Health Organisation (Europe Region), the International Agency for Research on Cancer and Europe Against Cancer. In it, tobacco production and use, the constituents of tobacco, and the relationship between tobacco and cancers are examined. No doubt is left as to the seriousness of the carcinogenic effects of tobacco. The message is tersely and effectively summarized in the title of the booklet from which the paper was drawn: *Tobacco or Health.*

Passive smoking has recently been recognized as a real threat to non-smokers who may acquire lung cancer and many other diseases as a result of breathing in the smoke of others. Passive smoking appears to be especially harmful to small babies, to young children and to those who are already suffering from a variety of illnesses. In the paper 'Passive smoking', Martin Jarvis summarizes the evidence for the harmful effects of inhaling

other people's smoke. The risks of passive smoking are far greater than those posed by any other indoor man-made pollutant. Jarvis discusses the implications that this information has for employers, people in charge of public places, health care professionals and for legislators in whose power it is to bring about legislation to protect the rights of every citizen to breathe smoke-free air. The issue of passive smoking introduces important extra ammunition for people who want to control the epidemics that are brought about by tobacco consumption.

Reference

Pott, P. (1775) *Chirurgical observations relative to the cataract, the polypus of the nose, the cancer of the scrotum, the different kinds of ruptures, and the mortification of the toes and feet*, Havers, Clarke and Collins, London, 63–65.

NUTRITION AND PREVENTION OF HUMAN CANCER

Michael Hill

Introduction

In this paper, the questions to be answered are:

(a) What is the evidence relating nutrition to cancer risk?

(b) Why is it so difficult to carry out research in this field and to interpret the data?

(c) What is the relative importance of micronutrients (trace elements, vitamins etc.) compared with macronutrients (fat, protein, fibre)?

(d) What is the relative importance of food additives and contaminants?

(e) On the basis of the above, what dietary advice can be given and with what level of confidence?

These questions will be dealt with in turn.

What is the evidence relating nutrition to cancer risk?

The evidence relating nutrition to cancer risk is derived principally from two sources, namely animal studies and human epidemiology. This is supported, in the case of certain cancer sites, by postulated mechanisms, amenable to investigation, that add plausibility to the proposed relationships.

Animal studies

The earliest animal experiments were carried out by Tannenbaum (1945) and Tannenbaum and Silverstone (1953) who showed that when rodents were fed a calorie-restricted diet in comparison with controls fed *ad libitum*, they were not only slimmer and much more lively and active, but they also had a much longer life span and a very much lower risk of spontaneous tumour formation. These results

have been repeated, extended and confirmed by many groups in subsequent years (Tucker, 1979; Kritchevsky *et al.*, 1986) and could imply a relation between cancer risk and total energy intake or intake of fat or protein, or with some factors secondarily related to diet.

In addition, there is now a vast body of experimental data relating the intake of dietary fat to the risk of induced cancers of the breast (Carroll, 1985; Dao and Chan, 1983) and large bowel (Nigro *et al.*, 1975; Reddy *et al.*, 1976) and more limited data for other cancer sites (e.g. uterus, prostate, pancreas). Other studies have shown protective effects of dietary fibre in colorectal cancer (Freeman *et al.*, 1984), beta-carotene in the later stages of experimental gastric cancer, vitamins C and E in nitrosamine-induced cancers and so on. This experimental evidence has been summarized recently in numerous reviews (Kritchevsky *et al.*, 1986; Carroll, 1985; Nigro, 1986a, 1986b; Hill, 1986a).

As with much scientific observation, there has been a body of contradictory evidence. Much ingenuity has been shown in intended experiments designed to reveal whether the apparent relation between diet/nutrition and risk of cancer is causally or coincidentally related to diet. This has proved to be very much simpler in the animal studies than in human work. It must now be accepted as proven.

For example, there has been dispute concerning the role of fat. Where all other diet components remain constant, then an increase in fat also increases the energy content of the diet. However, for example with colorectal cancer, in isocaloric diets, unsaturated fats 'cause' more tumours than do saturated fats (Sakaguchi *et al.*, 1986), and trans fatty acids 'cause' more tumours than do cis fatty acids (Reddy *et al.*, 1985); in such studies, all other dietary components can be standardized and only the type of fat changes, making it difficult to dispute the role of specific types of fat. In other experiments, the amount of fat is increased and the diets kept isocaloric by varying the amount of some other energy source, such as simple starches or oligasaccharide. Such experiments confirm the dose–response relationship between fat intake and cancer risk in such models (Reddy *et al.*, 1985).

Human epidemiological studies

Epidemiological investigations into the relationship between diet, nutrition and cancer risk can be divided into three classes, namely international correlations (also termed ecological studies), case-control studies and prospective studies. These are best illustrated using colorectal cancer as an example, but there is a similar body of evidence relating diet to breast cancer, a large body for endometrial cancer and numerous reports for other cancer sites.

There have been very many international correlation studies relating diet/nutrition to colorectal cancer risk, and these are summarized in Table 1. Where all dietary factors are considered, almost all such studies show a very strong correlation with the amount of dietary fat or meat (Armstrong and Doll, 1975; Drasar and Irving, 1973; Gregor *et al.*, 1969; Liu *et al.*, 1979; Eyssen, 1984). With rather less unanimity they tend also to show an inverse correlation with dietary fibre (Liu *et al.*, 1979; Eyssen, 1984). The correlations with animal fat tend to be much stronger than those with plant (Armstrong and Doll, 1975; Drasar and Irving, 1973).

Table 1 International correlation studies relating diet to colorectal cancer and to breast cancer

Number of countries compared	Observation	Reference
Colorectal cancer		
23	Strong correlation with fat and meat	Armstrong and Doll, 1975
37	Strong correlation with fat and meat; none with dietary fibre	Draser and Irving, 1973
28	Strong correlation with animal protein	Gregor *et al.* 1969
47	Correlation of rectal cancer with beer consumption	Enstom, 1977
20	Correlation with fat and (inversely) with fibre	Liu *et al.* 1979
25	Correlation with fat and (inversely) with fibre	Eyssen and Bright-See, 1984
Breast cancer		
37	Strong correlation with dietary fibre	Draser and Irving, 1973
25	Strong correlation with dietary fibre	Carroll, 1985

A major criticism of the ecological studies is that the populations compared differ in many ways as well as in diet. For this reason, the results of case-control studies, where the controls are matched to the cases as closely as possible to prevent coincidental correlations emerging, are preferred by epidemiologists. There have been many such studies and their results have been very much less clear cut than have those of the ecological studies. Nevertheless, many of them, particularly the more recent reports (Jain *et al.*, 1980; Potter and McMichael, 1986; Kune and Kune, 1987), show a correlation with the intake of meat or fat and (inversely) with dietary fibre.

The most reliable results are obtained from prospective studies, in which the diet of large numbers of individuals are determined and the populations then followed to see which of them develops the disease being studied. There have been few such studies. The biggest – a follow-up of more than 250,000 Japanese by Hirayama (1981) – has produced evidence in favour of a role for meat and fat in colorectal carcinogenesis and a major protective role for green leafy vegetables. The role for fat and meat was further supported in a prospective study by Willett *et al.* (1990).

Mechanisms

A major reason for believing that the relationship between diet and cancer risk is causal and not coincidental is that mechanisms have been proposed which make such relationships plausible (Hill and Thompson, 1984; Hill, 1987). Thus, in colorectal carcinogenesis, it has been proposed that increased dietary fat and meat and decreased dietary fibre cause an increased faecal concentration of bile acids (Hill, 1986; Hill, 1989b). These latter have been shown to be potent tumour promoters and to increase the rate of adenoma growth. This proposed mechanism is amenable to testing, and has survived such testing very well.

Many breast and all endometrial cancers are oestrogen dependent. Dietary fat is known to increase both the concentration of circulating oestrogen and, by increasing the amount of tissue adiposity, the concentration of oestrogen receptors in both the breast and the endometrium (Hill and Thompson, 1984; Hill, 1987). Again, this hypothesis has been extensively tested and has stood up well to such examination.

When an observed relationship can be explained by a postulated mechanism, when that mechanism is subjected to rigorous examination and survives, this lends considerable credibility to the initial observation. Some of these proposed mechanisms have been summarized recently by Hill (Hill and Thompson, 1984; Hill, 1987).

Why is it so difficult to investigate this field?

In one respect the preceding section has been misleading – in only giving the final conclusions.

In the field of human epidemiology, by far the strongest correlations have been obtained by **comparing populations**, but these studies can be subjected to considerable criticism. First, the data used in such correlations are the cancer incidences and the nutritional intakes of populations. Cancer incidence data are usually collected for certain defined areas of regions which rarely cover the whole of a country. Nutritional data are collected by WHO and are usually for specific regions that rarely correspond to those for which the cancer statistics apply. Further, the food *intake* data are in fact normally based only on food *sold* in shops (ignoring, for example, home-grown vegetables) and take no account of food wastages, etc. It is clear that the data available are not ideal and must therefore be treated with caution. In addition, the populations compared may differ in many respects other than diet; these differences include genetic, environmental, climatic, socio-economic and geographical factors.

All of these criticisms can be met by using **case-control studies,** where the cases can be matched closely to the controls. However, case-control studies have their own drawbacks. Loss of appetite is a common feature of serious illness and this must be taken into account for the cases, but not the controls. To obviate these problems, it is common to attempt to determine the diet consumed before the onset of symptoms and this necessitates the use of diet-recall methods. These methods are notoriously inaccurate, and yield data that are not very reliable. In addition, although it is possible to match cases to controls in order to screen out coincidental correlations, assumptions must be made about the causation of the disease in order to determine which factors need to be controlled.

The ideal type of epidemiological study is the **prospective study**; in this type of approach, the current diet is determined in a group of normally healthy persons (a relatively accurate procedure) and the cohort is then followed for many years to see which people go on to develop cancer. The major problems with such an approach are the numbers of people needed, the length of follow-up needed, and the need to monitor the cohort during the follow-up. (In a prospective study of colorectal cancer in the UK, a population of 8,000 persons aged 45 to 75 needed to be followed for 10 years in order to yield 50 cases of the disease.) Normally in a case-control study, it is usual to accumulate 200 to 500 cases, and the determination of the diet of such a group and their controls (normally by means of an administered questionnaire lasting two to four hours) is manageable.

In contrast, the effort required to determine the diet of the tens of thousands of persons needed in a good prospective study is a major undertaking. During the follow-up period, the cohort must be monitored in case of changes in diet (as a result, for example, of health campaigns) and in a long follow-up it may be necessary to make more than one assessment of diet. Such studies are usually regarded as prohibitively expensive unless there is very

good evidence already available to support the hypothesis tested. The length of follow-up necessary before results are available is also a major problem with such studies.

Because of all of these problems, it is only recently that a degree of consensus has been reached in the epidemiological studies. In colorectal cancer, a number of recent case-control studies (designed to avoid the problems cited above) have yielded results in agreement with the international correlations and showing a correlation with fat and meat intake. Similar recent case-control studies of breast cancer have shown correlations with intake of animal fat, in agreement with the International correlations.

Because of the problems with epidemiological studies, many groups have turned to **animal experimentation** as a means of resolving the situation. In animal experiments, the test animals can easily be made genetically homogenous, housed under identical conditions and fed defined diets in defined amounts. Despite this, the contribution to our understanding of the relation between diet and cancer risk from animal studies has been very disappointing. In breast cancer, the animal experiments, whilst indicating a clear role for fat, suggest that unsaturated fats pose a greater risk than saturated fats, in contrast to the human disease. Similarly, in experimental colorectal cancer, the role of dietary fibre is extremely confused. Criticisms of the animal studies have been summarized by Hill (1989c).

Role of trace elements, vitamins and precursors

The vast bulk of evidence relating diet and nutrition to the risk of human cancer concerns the macronutrients (fat in cancer of the breast, colon and endometrium; poor nutrition in cancer of the oesophagus and stomach; alcohol in cancer of the oesophagus, rectum and liver) but there is evidence for a role for trace elements and micronutrients. The evidence suggests a relatively minor role for such micronutrients. The scientific background to the role of micronutrients has been reviewed recently by Diplock (1988).

Trace elements

The trace element that has received most attention has been selenium. A number of studies have shown lower serum selenium concentrations in cancer cases than in control persons for certain cancers. The cancer sites most commonly cited are in the digestive tract. The most serious criticism of these results is the known avidity of tumours for selenium, which suggests that the low serum selenium levels in cancer cases may be due to scavenging of the selenium. In some animal studies, the amount of selenium in the tumours could account almost totally for the decreased serum level. Selenites have antioxidant properties that have been postulated to be responsible for any protective effect.

Vitamins

The vitamins most commonly mentioned in this context are vitamins A, C and E.

Vitamin A (retinol) has been claimed to be protective against cancer of the lung and of the oropharynx. A very large study was carried out in Brazil (the 'Brazilian red oil' study) to substantiate this but unfortunately those using the red oil (very rich in retinol) had the same cancer risk as those who did not use the red oil. The study has been reported, but not published.

Vitamin C has been shown by many groups to be associated with a decreased risk of gastric cancer (Gey *et al.*, 1987). It has been postulated that the mechanism of this protective effect is through the ability of ascorbic acid to scavenge nitrite and so prevent the formation of carcinogenic nitrosamines (Reed *et al.*, 1983). This is under investigation by a number of groups.

Vitamin E has anti-oxidant properties in the lipid phase and should therefore be a

scavenger of proximate carcinogens in the tissues. There is some evidence from epidemiology to support this, but it is insufficient to justify dietary recommendations with respect to this vitamin.

Precursors

The major precursor discussed in the context of cancer risk is beta-carotene – a retinol precursor. In many, usually American, studies (Gey *et al.*, 1987; Merkes *et al.*, 1986) beta-carotene has been implicated as protecting against gastric carcinogenesis – a role that appears to be taken by ascorbic acid in European studies. This is being further investigated by South American groups, and the results of these projects are awaited with interest. A more general role for beta-carotene in cancer prevention has been proposed, particularly with respect to lung cancer (Temple and Basu, 1988).

Conclusion

There is some evidence implicating trace elements, vitamins and precursors. However, even if the most favourable results obtained so far can be confirmed, the prospects for cancer prevention by means of adequate micronutrient intake are of minor importance in comparison with the potential effect of the macronutrients.

What is the role of food additives and contaminants?

The evidence available at present indicates that the number of cancers possibly caused by food additives is very tiny in comparison with the number caused by the macronutrients, or even the micronutrients. The importance of preservatives (such as nitrite) as antioxidants on food quality and public health is such that there should be no question of, for example, risking botulism by banning nitrite as a food additive (although the position of food colours is difficult to justify).

The most important food contaminants with respect to cancer risk are the mycotoxins (such as aflatoxin) caused by fungal contamination. In many parts of the world aflatoxin is thought to be a major risk factor in hepatic cancer (Wogan, 1975) in conjunction with hepatitis B virus infection. In western populations this is not an important risk factor because the climate is less favourable to fungal food spoilage, and because food storage technology is capable of controlling this risk.

What dietary advice can be given and with what confidence?

Of the factors considered above, clearly the major risk is associated with macronutrients; however, a change in one macronutrient *must* be associated with counter changes in the other macronutrients. In contrast, micronutrients, food additives and contaminants can be modulated in isolation.

There can be no dispute that fungal contaminated food must be avoided and, if necessary, appropriate food additives used to prevent such contamination. This would, however, have little effect on the current cancer risk in western populations and would be more important as a means of preventing than of solving a problem.

There can also be little dispute that fresh fruit and salad type vegetables are an important source of vitamins and micronutrients. There have been no major reports claiming any deleterious effect on cancer or other health risk of such fresh foods. Thus, although this is unlikely to have a major impact on the cancer incidence in western countries, it will have some beneficial effect and no known drawbacks.

The problems arise with the advice to be given on the intake of macronutrients. In affluent western societies, diet is a matter of choice and the foods that people eat are chosen for palatability as well as for health aspects. If we

recommend changes in the macro diet, we must accept, therefore, that we are probably asking people to eat a diet that they regard as less palatable than that which would be otherwise chosen. The lifetime risk of, for example, colorectal cancer is about 5%, which means that 95% of people will *not* get the disease.

It is apparent that well-fed healthy western peoples are more resistant to virus and bacterial infections. Influenza had a 20% mortality in Glasgow shortly after World War I and this has been ascribed to the poor nutritional status of that population; very few die of the disease now. Similarly, diseases such as scarlet fever and childhood mumps generate few fears in comparison with the 1920s (when both caused many deaths). Thus, when we ask people to change their macro-diet, we must consider that not only were 95% not going to get the disease in the first place, but that we may unwittingly increase the risk of reducing resistance to other disease.

In consequence, there is a body of opinion that believes that we need to be very sure of the benefits and very sure of lack of adverse 'side effects' before we make such recommendations to the general public.

In recent years, the evidence in favour of decreasing the amount of dietary fat in order to decrease the risk of heart disease, cancers of the large bowel, breast and endometrium, as well as obesity-related diseases, has probably reached the level needed to convince an informed public. Similarly, an increased intake of dietary fibre is probably justified for reasons of improved colonic physiology and its likely effect on constipation and diverticular disease (Eastwood *et al.*, 1978), to which can be added a possible beneficial effect on the risk of colorectal cancer (Jensen, 1989). The concern here is the risk of increasing the prevalence of symptoms of food sensitivity and irritable bowel syndrome (Alun Jones *et al.*, 1982, 1985; Hunter *et al.*, 1985).

In contrast to the doubts that many have about advice to the whole population, there are few doubts about the value of advice to sub-populations known to be at high risk of diet-related cancer. Such groups include close relatives of cancer cases and special patient groups where the increased risk is great enough to make the risk of side effects less likely to adversely affect the cost-benefit analysis of such advice.

Conclusions

According to a number of analyses, 30 to 40% of cancers in western populations have a dietary etiology. We are making considerable headway in determining the specific dietary items causing this relationship and a diet rich in fat or meat and low on fresh fruits, salads and cereal-based foods appears to confer an increased risk of cancer. However, it is essential that the risk of cancer should not be studied in isolation but should be seen as part of an overall attack on chronic disease of all types.

References

Alun Jones, V., Dickinson, R.J., Workman, E. *et al.* (1985) Crohn's disease: maintenance of remission by diet, *Lancet* **2**, 177–180.

Alun Jones, V., McLaughlin, P., Shorthouse, M. *et al.* (1982) Food intolerance: a major factor in the pathogenesis of irritable bowel syndrome, *Lancet* **2**, 1115–1117.

Armstrong, B. and Doll, R. (1975) Environmental factors and cancer incidence and mortality in different countries with special reference to dietary practices, *Int. J. Cancer* **15**, 617–631.

Carroll, K.K. (1985) Diet and breast cancer: experimental approaches. In Joosens, J., Hill, M. and Geboers, J. (eds.) Diet and human carcinogenesis, *Excerpta Medica*, Amsterdam, 265–273.

Dao, T.L. and Chan P.C. (1983) Effect of duration of high fat intake on enhancement of mammary carcinogenesis in rats, *J. Natl. Cancer Inst.* **71**, 201–205.

Diplock, A.T. (1988) Micronutrients and trace elements in cancer prevention, In Reed, P. and Hill, M. (eds.) Gastric carcinogenesis, *Excerpta Medica*, Amsterdam, 99–104.

Drasar, B.S. and Irving, D. (1973) Environmental factors and cancer of the colon and breast, *Br. J. Cancer* **27**, 167–172.

Eastwood, M.A., Smith, A.N., Boydon, W.G. *et al.* (1978) A comparison of bran ispaghula and lactose on colon function in diverticular disease, *Gut* **19**, 1144–1147.

Eyssen, G.E. and Bright-See, E. (1984) Dietary factors in colon cancer: international relationships, *Nutr. Cancer* **6**, 160–170.

Freeman, H.J., Spiller, G.A. and Kim, Y.S. (1984) Effect of high hemicellulose corn bran in 1,2-dimethyl hydrazine-induced rat intestinal neoplasia, *Carcinogenesis* **5**, 261–264.

Gey, K.F., Brubacher, G.B. and Stahelin, H.B. (1987) *Am. J. Clin. Nutr.* **45**, 1368–1377.

Gregor, O., Toman, R. and Prusova, F. (1969) Gastrointestinal cancer and nutrition, *Gut* **10**, 1031–1034.

Hill, M.J. (1986) Biochemical approaches to the prevention of colorectal cancer, *Prog. Clin. Biol. Res.* **186**, 263–276.

Hill, M.J. (1987) Dietary fat and human cancer, *Anticancer Res.* **7**, 281–292.

Hill, M.J. (1989a) Experimental studies of fat, fibre and calories. In Miller, A.B. (ed.) *Diet and aetiology of cancer*, Springer, Heidelberg, 31–38.

Hill, M.J. (1989b) The mechanism of carcinogenesis in the gastrointestinal tract, *Verh. Bd.* **24**, 141–146.

Hill, M.J. (1989c) Experimental studies of fat, fibre and calories in carcinogenesis. In Miller, A.B. (ed.) *Diet and the aetiology of cancer*, Springer, Heidelberg, 31–38.

Hill, M.J. and Thompson, M.H. (1984) Role of endogenous carcinogens. In Stroll, B. (ed.) *Risk factors and multiple cancer*, Wiley, London, 103–132.

Hirayama, T. (1981) A large scale cohort study on the relation between diet and selected cancers of digestive organs, In Bruce *et al.* (eds.) *Gastrointestinal cancer: endogenous factors*, Cold Spring Harbour Lab Press, New York, 409–429.

Hunter, J.O., Workman, E. and Alun Jones, V. (1985) The role of diet in the management of irritable bowel syndrome, *Topics on Gastroenterology* 12, 305–313.

Jain, M., Cook, G.M., Davis, F.G. *et al.* A case-control study of diet and colorectal cancer, *Int. J. Cancer* 26, 757–768.

Jensen, O.M. (1989) Dietary fibre, carbohydrate and cancer: epidemiological evidence. In Miller, A.B. (ed.) *Diet and the aetiology of cancer*, Springer, Heidelberg, 21–30.

Kritchevsky, D., Weber, M.M., Buck, C.L.and Klurfield, D.M. (1986) Calories, fat and cancer, *Lipids* 21, 272–274.

Kune, G.A.and Kune, S. (1987) The nutritional causes of colorectal cancer: an introduction to the Melbourne study, *Nutr. Cancer* 9, 1–4.

Liu, K., Stamler, J., Moss, D. *et al.* Dietary cholesterol, fat and fibre and colon cancer mortality, *Lancet* 2, 782–785.

Merkes, M.S., Comstock, G.W., Villeumier, J.P., *et al.* (1986) *New Engl. J. Med.* 315, 1250–1254.

Nigro, N. (1986a) Animal experimentation and prevention of colorectal cancer, In Vahouny, G. and Kritchevsky, D. (eds.), *Dietary fiber*, Plenum, New York, 481–485.

Nigro, N. (1986b) Animal models of colorectal cancer, *Prog. Clin. Biol. Res.* 186, 161–174.

Nigro, N., Singh, D.V., Campbell, R.L. and Pak M.S. (1975) Effects of dietary beef fat on intestinal tumour formation by azoxymethane in rats, *J. Natl. Cancer Inst.* 54, 439–442.

Potter, J. and McMichael, A. (1986) Diet and cancer of the colon and rectum : a case-control study, *J. Natl. Cancer* Inst. 76, 577–569.

Reddy, B.S., Narisawa, T., Vukusich, D., Weisburger, J.H. and Wynder, E.L. (1976) Effect of quantity and quality of dietary fat and dimethyl hydrazine in colon carcinogenesis in rats, *Proc. Soc. Exp. Biol. Med.* 151, 237–239.

Reddy, B.S., Tanaka, T. and Simi, B. (1985) Effect of different levels of dietary trans fat or corn oil on azoxymethane-induced colon carcinogenesis in F344 rats, *J. Natl. Cancer Inst.* 75, 791–798.

Reed, P.I., Summers, K., Smith, P.L.R., *et al.* (1983) *Gut* 24, 492–493.

Sakaguchi, M., Minoura, T. and Hiramatsu, Y. *et al.* (1986) Effect of dietary saturated and unsaturated fatty acids on faecal bile acids and colon carcinogenesis induced by azoxymethane in rats, *Cancer Res.* 46, 61–65.

Tannenbaum A. (1945) The dependence of tumour formation on the degree of caloric restriction, *Cancer Res.* 5, 609–615.

Tannenbaum A. and Silverstone, J. (1953) Nutrition in relation to cancer, *Adv. Cancer Res.* 1, 451–501.

Temple, N.J., Basu, T.K. (1988) Does beta-carotene prevent cancer? A critical review, *Nutr. Res.* 8, 685–701.

Tucker M.J. (1979) The effect of long-term food restriction on tumours in rodents. *Int. J. Cancer* 23, 803–807.

Willett, W.C., Stampfer, M.J., Colditz, G.A. *et al.* Relation of meat, fat and fibre intake to the risk of colon cancer in a prospective study among women, *New Engl. J. Med.* 323, 1664–1672.

Wogan, G.N. (1975) Dietary factors and special epidemiological situations of liver cancer in Thailand and Africa, *Cancer Res.* 35, 3499–3502.

Recommended reading list

Miller, A.B. (ed.) (1989) *Diet and the aetiology of cancer*, Springer, Heidelberg.

Joosens, J., Hill, M. and Geboers, J. (eds.) (1985) Diet and human carcinogenesis, *Excerpta Medica*, Amsterdam.

Hunter, J. and Alun Jones, V. (eds.) (1985) *Food and the gut*, Balliere-Tyndall, London.

Hill, M. and Giacosa, A. (eds.) (1991) *Causation and prevention of human cancer*, Kluwer, London.

Pekins, E. and Visek, W. (eds.) (1983) *Dietary fat and health*, AOCS, Illinois.

BNF Task Force (1990) *Complex carbohydrates in foods*, Chapman and Hall, London.

MALIGNANT MELANOMA – THE STORY UNFOLDS

Rona M. MacKie

The epidemiology of cutaneous malignant melanoma in Europe

Studies of the epidemiology of malignant melanoma in Europe have been carried out most extensively in Scandinavia, Germany and Great Britain.

The epidemiology of malignant melanoma in Scandinavia has been well studied over the past 20 years. In Norway, Magnus was one of the earliest to study melanoma epidemiology (Magnus, 1973, 1982). He clearly recognized, firstly, that the incidence of melanoma in Scandinavia was rising rapidly and, secondly, that there was a relationship between the incidence of melanoma and exposure to ultraviolet light. Magnus's work was carried out mainly with populations of patients with melanoma first registered in the 1960s and 1970s. He observed that the incidence of melanoma was doubling every 10 years.

He further recognized that there was what is known as a cohort effect. This term is used to define the observation that each group of individuals born in successive decades has a greater likelihood of developing the disease in question. Thus, the cohort of individuals born in the 1930s has a greater risk of developing melanoma than those born in the 1920s. This observation clearly implicates a change in the habits of whole populations which occurred at a fixed point in time rather than a sporadic behavioural change on the part of individuals.

Magnus's work pinpoints the likely change in habits to the mid-1930s. It was then that the change in attitude occurred with regard to the desirability of a suntan. Prior to this time, the fashionable skin colour was pale. Normal summer attire for women was a long dress, stockings and a parasol. Coco Chanel in France in the 1930s made a suntan fashionable. Very shortly thereafter, fashions changed dramatically with regard to beachwear and summer clothes. Arms, legs and parts of the trunk were exposed to summer sunlight, and bathing suits have steadily become briefer.

More recently in Scandinavia, the work of Østerlind and her colleagues in Denmark has contributed a great deal to our current understanding of cutaneous malignant melanoma. A study of malignant melanoma patients presenting in Denmark between the years 1978 and 1982 (Østerlind, 1988) shows an annual age-adjusted incident of 8.4 cases per 100,000 of the population in women and 6.1 cases per 100,000 of the population in men. This series shows that if we study age in relation to incidence of melanoma there is a steady increase in incidence rates from the teenage years up to the age of 35 to 45, when it levels off. Women are found to develop melanoma more frequently than men until the age of 80 years. Below the age of 40, twice as many women as men are affected by malignant melanoma. These observations contrast with Østerlind's study of basal cell carcinoma and squamous cell carcinoma in Denmark, where there is a steady increase with age, with the highest numbers found in the over-80 age group.

In Østerlind's study there are very striking and interesting differences in the sites which are affected by the different types of cutaneous malignancies. For melanoma, males are found to have the highest number on the back, with 19.5 cases occurring in every 100,000. The second most common site in men is the face, followed by the anterior chest. For women, the leg between the knee and the ankle is the most likely place, with 17.6 women per 100,000 developing melanoma on this site. The second most common site for women is the back and the third most common the face. Thus males have a higher incidence of melanoma above the waist, and females have a higher incidence of melanoma below the waist. When we compare these figures with those for basal cell carcinoma and squamous cell carcinoma there are again striking site-related differences. By far the commonest site for both basal and squamous cell carcinoma in both sexes is the face, scalp and neck.

A second study carried out by Østerlind (Østerlind *et al.*, 1988) in Denmark, looking at a case-control study of patients with cutaneous malignant melanoma, investigated the importance of exposure to ultraviolet radiation in patients who develop melanoma by comparison with an age- and sex-matched normal control group. A significantly increased risk of developing melanoma has been identified in those who developed severe sunburn before the age of 15 and in those who enjoyed sunbathing, boating and vacations in the sun as hobbies.

By contrast, however, there was a significantly decreased risk of developing melanoma amongst males who had an occupational exposure to sunlight during the summer months. In this particular study, no association was found between the risk of cutaneous malignant melanoma and exposure to any form of artificial ultraviolet radiation. Particular sources of radiation included in this study were fluorescent lighting, sun lamps and sunbeds. It must be noted, however, that the population was gathered between the years of 1982 and 1985. Prior to 1985, a very limited number of sunbeds of the modern type with the long UVA tubes were in use.

A case-controlled study carried out on a German population showed once again that patients who tan poorly and burn easily tend to be more at risk than those who tan easily and do not develop burning on exposure to ultraviolet radiation (Garbe *et al.*, 1989).

Figures for the United Kingdom also show a steady increase in incidence (OPCS). Incidence figures for 1984 for England and Wales show an incidence of 5.8 per 100,000 in women and 3.1 per 100,000 in men. This 2:1 female:male ratio is consistently found in studies carried out in both England and Wales and in Scotland. In other parts of Europe, there is a slight female preponderance, but this is most marked in the UK series. Looking at age-specific incidence, it will be found that there are very few melanomas registered prior to puberty, but that after the age range 15 to 24 the numbers rise steadily and age-specific incidence is in fact highest in those aged 75 and over, with an incidence of 12.1 per 100,000 for females and 9.7 per 100,000 for males. These figures, compared with those for 1974, show a doubling in incidence in England and Wales over a 10-year period.

Figures for Scotland collected by the Scottish Melanoma Group in the years 1979 to 1988 inclusive show an 80% rise over the period of study. Throughout the 10-year period of study conducted by the Scottish Melanoma Group there is, as with England and Wales, a consistent 2:1 female:male ratio.

Mortality data for malignant melanoma are less easy to obtain. Figures for England and Wales come from the Office of Population Censuses and Surveys for the year 1986 and show 595 deaths from melanoma amongst women and 445 deaths from melanoma amongst men. This gives a death rate per million of the population of 23 for women and 18 for men for the England and Wales population. Compared against the world standard population, this gives a death rate for both sexes of 14 per million. As with incidence, mortality from malignant melanoma in England and Wales is rising steeply. Mortality in 1986–1987 compared with mortality from melanoma in the years 1951–1954 shows an increase of 177% in women and 250% for men.

Phenotypic characteristics of the melanoma patient

There is strong epidemiological evidence to suggest that malignant melanoma is associated with white-skinned individuals who have a significant amount of intermittent exposure to natural sunlight. The intermittent nature of this exposure appears to be important as in both Europe and other parts of the world, notably Australia, it is observed that those who have an outdoor occupation frequently have slightly lower rates of melanoma than those who have an indoor occupation but an outdoor recreation. This contrasts with other forms of skin cancer where the highest rates are found with the highest cumulative lifetime incidence of ultraviolet exposure.

Case-control studies are being carried out in many parts of the world to identify those features found in patients with melanoma which are not found in age- and sex-matched normal control members of the population. Studies in Denmark looking at large numbers of patients with melanoma have shown that the most important risk factors in Scandinavia were the number of raised benign pigmented naevi or moles on the arms, the amount of freckling experienced by an individual, and fair hair versus dark brown or black hair (Østerlind et al., 1988). Each of these risk factors was independent of the other. In this particular study, skin colour, whether it was dark, medium or light Caucasian skin, eye colour, and both acute and chronic reactions to sunburn in terms of developing sunburn or a deep tan, were not found to be important significant variables.

In view of the higher incidence of melanoma in women than in men in Europe, specific hormonal factors have been investigated in women. The Danish study carefully investigated the possible role of the oral contraceptive and number of pregnancies on the risk of developing melanoma (Østerlind et al., 1988a). This study found no associated risk with use of the oral contraceptive or other hormonal preparations and no association between parity and melanoma. A further study carried out in Denmark looking at risk factors has reported that there is no association between diet, alcohol, smoking habits and the use of hair dyes and the relative risk of melanoma (Østerlind et al., 1988b).

Studies in Germany looking at characteristics of melanoma patients have reported that melanoma patients have significantly more benign melanocytic moles or naevi with a diameter equal to, or greater than, 2mm (Garbe et al., 1989). In this study, the average mole count for a melanoma patient was 53 compared with 18 benign small naevi found on control cases. For individuals who have 60 or more small melanocytic naevi there is a 15 times greater risk of developing melanoma compared with those who have 10 or less small naevi.

In addition to a risk associated with small benign melanocytic naevi, a great deal of work has been done recently on the association between so-called 'dysplastic' naevi or clinically atypical naevi and increased risk of melanoma. Clinically atypical naevi are benign moles which are greater than 5mm in diameter and have an irregular edge, irregular colour or associated inflammation. The pathological features associated with these clinically atypical naevi which allow one to use the term 'dysplastic naevus' are the subject of ongoing debate. However, it is generally agreed that there is a pathological pattern in these lesions which is an intermediate stage between a totally benign melanocytic naevus and an early malignant melanoma.

In the German study, the presence of clinically atypical naevi was associated with a seven-times-greater risk of developing melanoma. In this German study, in contrast to the Scandinavian study, it was found that a lack of ability to tan was a significantly associated risk factor, with a relative risk of 2. No significant association was found between hair colour, eye colour and number of sunburns in the German study.

In a study carried out in Scotland, a significant association was reported between episodes of severe sunburn five years or less prior to development of the malignant melanoma (MacKie and Aitchinson, 1982). Patients with melanoma gave a history of such episodes three times more frequently than an age- and sex-matched control group. Also in Scotland it was found, as with Scandinavia and Germany, that large numbers of small benign melanocytic naevi were an extremely strong risk factor for malignant melanoma, and in the Scottish series were by far the strongest risk factor identified (Swerdlow *et al.*, 1986). In addition, in Scottish studies it has been shown that the presence of clinically atypical naevi as defined above and also the presence of freckles are independent risk factors for melanoma (MacKie *et al.*, 1989).

What triggers malignant melanoma, when and why?

There is strong epidemiological and case-control evidence to incriminate acute intermittent sun exposure in the aetiology of malignant melanoma. When ultraviolet radiation strikes the skin, damage is done to the nuclei of the individual cells. Free radicals are generated and minor abnormalities of DNA synthesis may occur. As a result of this ultraviolet stimulation, the body mobilizes DNA repair systems. The human cells in all parts of the body are continually going through a process of scheduled DNA repair which is associated with normal cell division and replacement of cells. The type of DNA repair that is carried out on the skin surface after ultraviolet radiation is termed unscheduled DNA repair.

There are several different types of unscheduled DNA repair, and one particular rare clinical disorder known as xeroderma pigmentosum is characterized by very poor unscheduled DNA repair after ultraviolet exposure on the part of the patients who have this disorder. These patients present clinically with early sunburn and skin damage, usually apparent by the age of one year, and go on to develop all types of skin cancer including melanoma in their early teens if they are not rigorously protected from strong sunlight.

This disease suggests that, without DNA repair mechanisms brought into play after ultraviolet light exposure, the incidence of melanoma would be higher. The assumption in the case of melanoma is that while a large number of benign melanocytes found in the basal layer of the epidermis do perform this function of unscheduled DNA repair satisfactorily, in time, one or two melanocytes do not perform this function perfectly. Because of the resulting abnormality in DNA synthesis, abnormal melanocytes are formed and the development of a clone of malignant melanoma cells is facilitated.

Ultraviolet radiation, when given to experimental animals, has, in addition to its carcinogenic effect, an effect on the body's immune system. When experimental mice are exposed to very high levels of ultraviolet radiation in the medium wavelength or UVB range similar to that found mainly in natural sunlight, a striking reduction in the body's immune system's capacity is noted. Studies carried out in man are not extensive, but do suggest that a mild degree of immunosuppression is also observed in humans after exposure to both natural sunlight and the ultraviolet radiation from solaria.

It is possible that this temporary reduction in the body's immune system's capacity may be associated with the development of malignancy. If the body's immune system is temporarily depressed, it may not be possible for the body to perform its normal function of immune surveillance and identify and remove an abnormally developing clone of cells. Thus the role of ultraviolet radiation may be two-fold, one in initiating cellular change which causes the melanocyte to transform from the benign to the malignant state and the second in allowing a temporary period of immunosuppression which makes the first event less likely to be identified and eliminated.

Changes in habits leading to greater sun exposure

Since the 1930s it has become increasingly fashionable to have a year-round sun tan. It is now quite acceptable for the great majority of the body surface area to be exposed to natural sunlight when the ambient temperature allows, and modern swim and sunbathing wear can be very brief.

In Northern Europe, such exposure could be of limited significance in view of the fact that the summer months and hours of sunlight are relatively short. However, this cosmetic desirability for a suntan and change in clothing fashions was followed in the 1950s with very much greater access to the Mediterranean beaches from the Northern European countries. Prior to 1950 air travel was limited in its availability by both price and number of flights. Since this time the introduction of the package holiday and charter flights have brought holidays on the Mediterranean coasts within the reach of the great majority of Northern Europeans. Norwegian studies have shown that melanoma patients have on average spent longer periods and larger numbers of holidays on the Mediterranean or similar coasts.

However, it must not be assumed that only Mediterranean sunlight can be responsible for severe burning which can be associated with the development of malignant melanoma. In a Scottish study, it was observed that one-third of the 111 melanoma patients studied in detail had never left the United Kingdom (MacKie and Aitchinson, 1982). It must therefore be emphasized in public education that any type of strong sunlight can lead to burning of unacclimatized skin, and that in the months of June and July in particular, northern countries may enjoy long hours of sunlight allowing such burning to take place.

In considering the factors leading to greater sun exposure which is both directly and indirectly implicated in the aetiology both of melanoma and of other skin cancers, we must therefore consider the ease of access of the public to countries with long hours of strong sunlight, the time spent out of doors, the lack of shade available on many Mediterranean beaches, the type of clothing worn when on such beaches, and the fact that until 10 years ago available sunscreens were limited in their efficiency.

The more recent problem which has arisen with habits of exposure to ultraviolet radiation has been the introduction of the UVA tanning bed and the use of commercially available solaria. Long wavelength ultraviolet light in the 320 to 360 nanometre range is termed UVA. This type of ultraviolet radiation does not cause the acute redness and burning after excessive exposure such as is seen after the medium wavelength UVB, which is the main wavelength found in natural sunlight. The availability since the early 1980s of fluorescent tubes which emit predominantly UVA has led to the growth of the suntan parlour industry. Prospective clients are encouraged to believe that the acquisition of a UVA-induced tan in a tanning parlour can prepare their skin for natural summer sunshine and to take a course of UVA sun exposure prior to their annual holiday. Further encouragement is given to individuals to maintain a year-round tan by using the solaria two or three times a week during the winter months.

Sunbeds and sun canopies were initially mainly available in health clubs, in hairdressing salons and similar institutions. The recent reduction in the cost of these machines has rendered their availability for domestic use. Initially it was hoped because of the limited erythema and burning induced by UVA, that pure UVA would not be a cause of skin cancer. Unfortunately, work over the past decade has shown clearly that UVA alone is a cause of all types of skin cancer in animal models. Recent work from both Scotland (MacKie et al., 1989) and from a Canadian study (Walter et al., 1990) has further emphasized that the use of modern sunbeds emitting only UVA is also a risk factor for malignant melanoma.

Steps that can be taken to reduce the death rate from malignant melanoma

Two main approaches can be considered when contemplating programmes to reduce mortality from malignant melanoma. The first is the policy of **primary prevention**. This implies that we are aware of the cause of malignant melanoma and can encourage the public to take appropriate avoiding action so that they are not exposed to the cause.

The alternative approach is that of **secondary prevention**. This assumes that patients will continue to develop melanoma but encourages an approach that will lead to curative measures being easily available for all patients who develop melanoma, and also an approach which encourages those who develop melanoma to attend *early* for appropriate treatment of their melanomas at a time when such cure can be achieved.

The prospects for primary prevention of malignant melanoma are relatively poor. The model for this type of approach are the campaigns run over the past 20 to 30 years to reduce the incidence of lung cancer by discouraging cigarette smoking, and the results of such campaigns have been disappointing. Similarly, it will be difficult to completely eradicate the habit of sunbathing. For individuals who live in a country which for most of the year is relatively cool and has low hours of natural sunlight, the annual holiday with exposure to stronger sunlight is regarded as both therapeutic and relaxing. The approach will therefore have to be to encourage sensible sun exposure rather than to ban it completely. Public education measures should be taken to explain to the public that excessive sun exposure on white skin can lead to skin cancer. A more immediate approach is to warn the public that prior to the development of skin cancer, excessive hours of sun exposure can lead to premature ageing.

Other factors which should be introduced into a campaign for primary prevention must be, first, **information** on the strength of UVB radiation from the sun around noon and an encouragement to avoid sun exposure on Mediterranean beaches or their equivalent between the hours of 11 a.m. and 3 p.m. In sunnier countries this may involve rescheduling outdoor activities, such as summer sporting fixtures, for the evening when the sun is less intense. Second, the **provision of shade** by tree planting campaigns and programmes near beaches, swimming pools, public parks, etc. for those who will be out of doors during periods of intense sunshine. Third, the encouragement of **the use of appropriate clothing** to shield skin from strong sunlight. This is particularly important for young children whose skin burns easily. A loose cotton teeshirt and the use of a sunhat should be encouraged. Only then should the use of sunscreens be introduced.

Over the past decade sunscreens have improved greatly in their ability to screen out UVB radiation. At present sunscreens are less effective at screening out UVA radiation but as the main carcinogenic component of natural sunlight lies in the UVB part of the spectrum these available sunscreens are of considerable value. All sunscreens have a skin protection factor or SPF number applied to them (MacKie, 1987). This number is an indication of the increase in time which can be spent out of doors prior to any redness of the skin developing compared to what would have happened if the individual was not using the preparation. Thus a preparation with an SPF of 10 indicates that 10 times as long can now be spent out of doors as could have been with no sun preparation applied.

SPF numbers are an approximation at present, but with any one range of products the higher SPF number preparations will screen ultraviolet more effectively than the lower preparations. Individuals should be encouraged to use high SPF preparations on themselves and on their children at the beginning of a holiday and only slowly to reduce the SPF number of the preparation used as their skin acclimatizes to the sun. Governments could help in this respect by making available at moderate subsidies a large pack of an effective sunscreen marketed in a way that will appeal to both sexes and also to children. Although there are already moves in this area on the part of industry, many sun screening preparations still appeal predominantly to females and are regarded as a cosmetic rather than an essential item of skin care for all ages and both sexes.

A programme such as that outlined above has already been started in the state of Victoria, Australia, where the incidence of both melanoma and non-melanoma skin cancer is extremely high. The use of role models such as the life guards on the surf beaches in Australia to encourage a more sensible approach to sun exposure appears to have already been effective in that teenagers are seeking less intense sun exposure and realizing the long-term hazards to their skin. As yet, there is no change in the mortality from skin cancer, but in time it is anticipated that this will occur.

Secondary prevention of melanoma implies a continuing research programme to develop the most effective curative strategies for malignant melanoma. At present, melanoma is treated predominantly by surgical excision, and the use of chemotherapy and radiotherapy is disappointing. Newer and more effective chemotherapeutic agents with specificity for melanoma must therefore be developed for dealing with patients with advanced disease.

Until these are available, the alternative approach to secondary prevention is to encourage patients to recognize early melanoma and to attend for treatment at a stage when the prospects for cure are good. Melanoma which has only invaded a millimetre or less below the skin's surface has excellent prospects for long-term cure. As it is quite possible to recognize melanoma at this stage, further public education campaigns

must be developed illustrating clearly the features of early malignant melanoma and encouraging individuals to examine their own skin and the skin of their partners and family, and to seek medical advice immediately if they have a pigmented lesion which could be melanoma.

Clearly those whose advice is sought must be able to take appropriate action. In many parts of Europe, this individual will be a dermatologist or surgeon, and in the UK this will most commonly be the general practitioner. The medical profession must therefore be well informed about the features of early melanoma and be able to initiate rapid surgical treatment or biopsy and pathological examination to confirm the nature of worrying pigmented lesions.

Such secondary prevention activities have been carried out in Queensland, Australia for many years (MacKie, 1988). During the time of these campaigns, the incidence of melanoma has continued to rise, but the death rate has not risen in parallel with this rising incidence. The inference is therefore that although habits of sun exposure have not until recently been altered, the public are attending for treatment with lesions which are at an earlier growth state and can therefore be cured more easily.

Similarly, a public education campaign carried out in Scotland in 1985 was associated with a statistically significant fall in the average tumour thickness of melanomas in the whole of Scotland (Doherty and MacKie, 1988). This implies that public education can alert individuals to features of possible early melanoma. It remains to be seen whether or not these UK public education studies will be associated with a fall in mortality.

In the US, many states have held Skin Cancer Fairs annually since 1985. These involve a free skin examination service and advice on consulting an appropriate dermatologist or surgeon about any worrying pigmented lesion. Because of ethical considerations, no treatment is offered at these Skin Cancer Fairs, and it is therefore difficult to assess their true efficacy other than as excellent publicity vehicles. Those attending who have lesions which are thought to be melanoma or indeed other types of skin cancer are advised to seek help from their dermatologist or other medical advisor or, if they do not have such an advisor, are given a list of appropriate individuals. Follow-up studies have not been carried out in depth to confirm the exact proportion of those given this advice who then seek such advice and have the lesion excised.

A recent exercise in the Netherlands involved the availability on four popular beaches in the summer months of a caravan offering free examination and advice concerning skin cancer. Large numbers of individuals sought advice at this caravan and a significant number of both melanoma and non-melanoma skin cancers were identified. The publicity surrounding this free skin cancer advice caravan was also an extremely useful vehicle for public education. One melanoma was identified for every 500 people examined.

A number of individual states in the US are considering introducing legislation to control the use of UVA sunbeds. At present, the contribution of UVA to skin cancer in general and melanoma in particular is relatively small, but clearly with long-term use this pattern could change. It may therefore be necessary to introduce, or consider the introduction of, similar legislation in Europe.

Raising public awareness of early melanoma and of its features will, of course, be associated with a degree of anxiety and encourage self-referral with a wide range of benign pigmented lesions, some of which are not malignant melanoma. Experience in Scotland has shown that one melanoma is identified for every 20 non-melanoma pigmented lesions referred from family doctors to specialists for opinion. If a vigorous national melanoma early detection campaign were to be mounted, the consequence could be large numbers of the public seeking advice about quite banal non-malignant pigmented lesions on their skin.

It is white-skinned individuals who are at risk, and, as stated earlier, children very rarely develop melanoma. The highest risk group is those who already have a family history of melanoma. Amongst those who have no such history, those who have large numbers of benign naevi, who burn easily and tan poorly, who freckle and who are fair-skinned and blue-eyed are the target group.

Personal experience indicates that after any period of publicity about early detection of melanoma, there is a temporary rise in referrals for reassurance. If any co-ordinated national activity were planned, the availability of triage clinics would be essential. Such clinics would be staffed by doctors with experience in recognizing early melanoma, probably dermatologists. Large numbers of patients can be examined relatively rapidly at such a clinic and the aim would be to divide the population into three main groups.

First would be those who probably had early melanoma and required minor skin surgery and pathological confirmation that the lesion in question was melanoma. The second would be those who had no disturbing lesions on their skin who required reassurance and discharge. Even this group, however, are very susceptible to education about sensible habits of sun exposure and the availability of leaflets designed for primary prevention of skin cancer at the time they seek advice is well worthwhile.

The third group are those who do not have lesions that are probably early melanoma, but who are considered in the higher risk factor groups. At present there is some debate as to whether or not such individuals should be put on long-term surveillance. Our own observations over 10 years of surveillance of a large number of individuals at a pigmented lesion clinic in the West of Scotland would suggest that the number of melanomas that develop in this population is so small as to make surveillance clinics economically unjustified. Nevertheless, such individuals must be given clear advice on what to look for in the way of changes in pigmented lesions that could indicate early melanoma, and what action to take if they are concerned. Both they and their general practitioners must be given appropriate information.

The incidence of cutaneous malignant melanoma is rising very rapidly. The rate of mortality from malignant melanoma is also rising, but slightly less rapidly. Measures are urgently needed to encourage both primary and secondary prevention of malignant melanoma. Prospects for secondary prevention are good and there are indications from countries such as Australia that they can be successful. Primary prevention should also be developed and national campaigns may well be needed for this.

References

Doherty, V.R. and MacKie, R.M. (1988) Experience of a public education programme on early detection of cutaneous malignant melanoma, *Br. Med. J.* **297**, 388–391.

Garbe, C., Krüger, S., Stadler, R., Guggenmoos-Holzmann, I. and Orfanos, C.E. (1989) Markers and relative risk in a German population for developing malignant melanoma, *Int. J. Dermatol.* **28**, 517–523.

Garbe, C., Wiebelt, H. and Orfanos, C.E. (1989) Change of epidemiological characteristics of malignant melanoma during the years 1962–1972 and 1983–1986 in the Federal Republic of Germany, *Dermatologica* **178**, 131–135.

MacKie, R.M. (1987) Links between exposure to ultraviolet radiation and skin cancer, *J. Royal Coll. Phys. Lond.* **21**, 91–96.

MacKie, R.M. (1988) Clinical and histological evidence of an association between benign melanocytic naevi and malignant melanoma, in Elwood, J.M. (ed.) *Melanoma and naevi – pigment cell*, **Vol. 9**, S. Karger, Basel, 48–58.

MacKie, R.M. and Aitchinson, T.C. (1982) Severe sunburn and subsequent risk of primary malignant melanoma in Scotland, *Br. J. Cancer* **46**, 955–961.

MacKie, R.M., Fruedenberger, T. and Aitchinson, T.C. (1989) Personal risk-factor chart for cutaneous melanoma, *Lancet* **ii**, 487–490.

Magnus, K. (1973) Incidence of malignant melanoma of the skin in Norway, 1955–1970, *Cancer* **32**, 1275–1286.

Magnus, K. (ed.) (1982) *Trends in cancer incidence*, Hemisphere Publishing Corporation, Washington, D.C.

Office of Population Censuses and Surveys, Medical Statistics Division – published data on incidence and mortality from melanoma in England and Wales.

Østerlind, A., Hou-Jenson, K. and Jensen, O.M. (1988) Incidence of cutaneous malignant melanoma in Denmark 1978–1982. Anatomic site distribution, histologic types, and comparison with non-melanoma skin cancer, *Br. J. Cancer* **58**, 385–391.

Østerlind, A., Tucker, M.A., Hou-Jensen, K, et al. (1988) The Danish case-control study of cutaneous malignant melanoma. I. Importance of host factors, *Int. J. Cancer* **42**, 200–206.

Østerlind, A., Tucker, M.A., Stone, B.J. and Jenson, O.M. (1988a) The Danish case-control study of cutaneous malignant melanoma. II. Importance of UV-light exposure, *Int. J. Cancer* **42**, 319–324.

Østerlind, A., Tucker, M.A., Stone, B.J. and Jenson, O.M. (1988b) The Danish case-control study of cutaneous malignant melanoma. III. Hormonal and reproductive factors in women, *Int. J. Cancer* **42**, 821–824.

Østerlind, A., Tucker, M.A., Stone, B.J. and Jenson, O.M. (1988c) The Danish case-control study of cutaneous malignant melanoma. IV. No association with nutritional factors, alcohol, smoking or hair dyes, *Int. J. Cancer* **42**, 825–828.

Swerdlow, A.J., English, J., MacKie, R.M., O'Doherty, C.J., Hunter, J.A.A., Clark, J. and Hole, D.J. (1986) Benign melanocytic naevi as a risk factor for malignant melanoma, *Br. Med. J.* **292**, 1555–1559.

Walter, S.D., Marrett, L.D., From, L., Hertzman, C., Shannon, H.S. and Roy, P. (1990) Association of cutaneous malignant melanoma with the use of sunbeds and sunlamps, *Int. J. Epidemiology* **131**, 232–243.

OCCUPATIONAL CANCER PREVENTION

Harri Vainio

Summary

Studies of occupational cancer are particularly significant for primary prevention of cancer. Firstly, most cancers, once identified, can be prevented by reasonably simple means, without impinging on personal freedom. Secondly, the prevention of occupational cancers represents a saving of lives and the elimination of illness during the most active period of the lifespan. A third reason for investigating occupational cancers is that, in some cases, workers represent a particularly heavily exposed subgroup, and the occupational setting thus serves as a laboratory for the general environment. The protection of human health in the workplace should not depend solely on the epidemiological demonstration of existing risks; it is essential that results of predictive toxicology from long- and short-term laboratory studies also be used in the identification of possible carcinogenic risk factors.

Historical development of knowledge about occupational cancer

The occurrence of cancers as a consequence of occupational exposure was recognized after the discovery of skin cancers among chimney sweeps (Pott, 1775). From that time, skin cancer served as a focal point for research on cancer in the workplace, due to the visibility of the disease and the simplicity of a contact theory of causation. Nevertheless, a century separated Pott's description of skin cancer among chimney sweeps and the extension of such studies to coal-tar and mineral oils, and a further 50 years passed before the carcinogens responsible were isolated in the laboratory by Cook and his co-workers (Cook *et al.*, 1932).

The first clear record of an internal neoplasm caused by occupational exposure to a complex carcinogen was inferred from the pattern of illness among miners in Schneeberg and Joachimstal. This illness and the attribution of its causation to coal dust were described by Paracelsus and Agricola in the 16th century, but it was not until the 20th century that radioactivity was implicated as a causative agent.

The association of bladder cancer with certain occupational exposure provides a historical illustration of the scientific potential of the epidemiological study of a relatively small number of rare tumours in a limited population. In 1895, Rehn reported three urinary bladder cancers among 45 workers in a German aniline dye factory (Rehn, 1895). This observation led to similar studies in many other countries and, eventually, to the implication of aromatic amines as causative factors in human bladder cancer. The International Labour Office indicated as early as 1921 that beta-naphthylamine and benzidine were the responsible carcinogens (International Labour Office, 1921). Experimental evidence was provided only later, by Hueper and his associates, who induced bladder cancer in dogs by repeated subcutaneous injections of beta-naphthylamine (Hueper *et al.*, 1938).

Since these early findings, many more carcinogenic occupational exposures have been identified by epidemiological methods. Figure 1 illustrates the historical development of knowledge about causal relationships between environmental factors and cancer and shows that epidemiological evidence for the involvement of carcinogenic factors is increasing exponentially (MacLure and MacMahon, 1980).

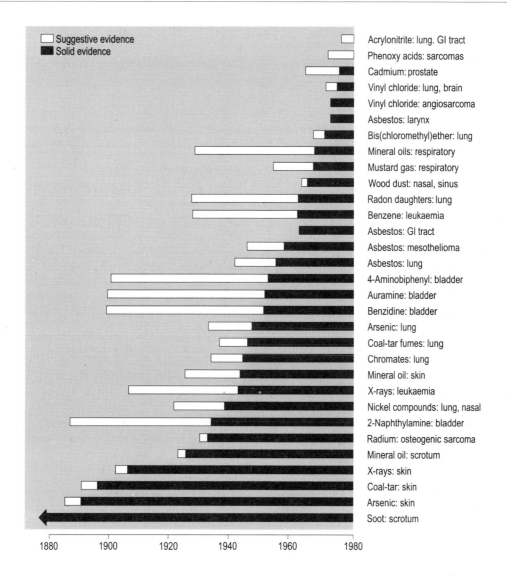

Figure 1 Occupational cancer: historical development of evidence

Importance of epidemiology in the identification of occupational carcinogens

To date, fewer that 20 specific substances encountered occupationally have been shown in epidemiological studies to be causally associated with cancer in humans (see Table 1). Eleven industrial processes are also known to entail exposures that are causally associated

with cancer formation (see Table 2). Table 3 lists all those industries and occupations that have been shown in epidemiological studies to be associated with increased risks of cancer, either causally or as a suspected association. This should by no means, however, be regarded as a complete list of the occupations in which exposures to carcinogens occur. For instance, evidence for the carcinogenicity of some compounds, such as alkylating anti-cancer drugs, has come from their use in therapy (see for example Schmähl and Kaldor, 1986); however, such compounds could also be carcinogenic through occupational exposure, and the potential hazards of these substances to hospital staff have recently been summarized elsewhere (Sorsa *et al.*, 1985).

Table 1 Chemicals and groups of chemicals causally associated with cancer in humans and to which the main type of exposure is of occupational origin

Exposure	Target organs[a]
4-Aminobiphenyl	Bladder
Arsenic and certain arsenic compounds	Skin, lung (liver, lymphatic and haematopoietic system)
Asbestos	Lung, pleura, peritoneum (gastrointestinal tract, larynx)
Benzene	Leukaemia
Benzidine	Bladder
Bis(chloromethyl)ether and technical-grade chloromethyl methyl ether	Lung
Chromium and certain chromium compounds	Lung (nasal cavity, gastrointestinal tract)
Coal-tars[b]	Skin
Coal-tar pitches	Skin (larynx, lung, oral cavity, bladder)
Erionite[c]	Pleura
Mineral oils (certain)	Skin (respiratory tract, bladder, gastrointestinal tract)
Mustard gas	Respiratory tract
beta-Naphthylamine	Bladder
Nickel and nickel compounds	Nasal sinus, lung (larynx)
Shale-oils	Skin (colon)
Soots	Skin, lung
Talc containing asbestiform fibres	Lung
Vinyl chloride	Liver (lung, brain, lymphatic and haematopoietic system, gastrointestinal tract

[a] Suspected associations are indicated in parentheses

[b] Iatrogenic exposures also

[c] Exposures mainly environmental in endemic areas

Source: Merletti *et al.*, 1984; IARC, 1987

Table 2 Industrial processes causally associated with cancer in humans

Exposure	Target organs[a]
Aluminium production	Lung
Auramine manufacture	Bladder
Boot and shoe manufacture and repair	Bone marrow, nasal sinus (bladder)
Coal gasification (older process)	Skin, lung (bladder)
Coke production	Skin, lung (kidney)
Furniture manufacture (wood dusts)	Nasal sinus
Isopropyl alcohol manufacture (strong acid process)	Nasal sinus (larynx)
Iron and steel founding	Lung
Magenta, manufacture of	Bladder
Rubber industry	Bladder, leukaemia (stomach, lung, skin)
Underground haematite mining (with exposure to radon)	Lung

[a] Suspected associations are indicated in parentheses

Source: IARC, 1987; Vainio et al., 1985

Table 3 Occupations involving exposure to chemicals, groups of chemicals, and industrial processes of complex mixtures for which there is sufficient evidence of carcinogenicity to humans

Industry	Occupation	Cancer site	Substance reported or suspected to be the causative agent	IARC Monographs reference
Agriculture, forestry and fishing	Arsenical insecticide application in vineyards	Lung, skin	Arsenic	23 (1980a)
Mining	Arsenic mining	Lung, skin	Arsenic	23 (1980a)
	Asbestos mining	Lung, pleural and peritoneal mesothelioma	Asbestos	14 (1977)
	Uranium and haematite mining	Lung	Radon daughters	-
Asbestos production	Insulating material production (pipes, sheeting, textile, clothes, masks, asbestos cement products)	Lung, pleural and peritoneal mesothelioma	Asbestos	14 (1977)

Petroleum industry	Shale-oil production	Skin, scrotum	Polynuclear aromatic hydrocarbons	35(1985)
Metal industry	Copper smelting	Lung	Arsenic	23 (1980a)
	Chromate production	Lung	Chromium	23 (1980a)
	Chromate plating	Lung	Chromium	23(1980a)
	Ferrochromium production	Lung	Chromium	23 (1980a)
	Nickel refining	Nasal sinuses, lung	Nickel	11 (1976)
	Metal machining	Skin	Mineral oils (containing various additives and impurities)	33 (1984a)
Ship building, motor vehicles and transport	Ship yard and dock yard work	Lung, pleural and peritoneal mesothelioma	Asbestos	14 (1977)
Chemical industry	Bis(chloromethyl)ether (BOME) and chloromethyl methyl ether (CMME) production and use	Lung (oatcell carcinoma)	BOME, CMME	4 (1974)
	Vinyl chloride producers	Liver angiosarcoma	Vinyl chloride monomer	19 (1979)
	Isopropyl alcohol manufacture (strong acid process)	Paranasal sinuses	Not identified	15 (1977)
	Pigment chromate production	Lung	Chromium	23 (1980a)
	Dye manufacture and use	Bladder	Benzidine, beta-naphthylamine, 4-aminobiphenyl	29 (1982b), 4 (1974), 1 (1972)
	Auramine manufacture	Bladder	Auramine (and other aromatic amines used in the process)	1 (1972)
Pesticides and herbicides production industry	Arsenical insecticides production and packaging	Lung	Arsenic	23 (1980a)

Gas industry	Coke plant work	Lung	Polycyclic aromatic hydrocarbons	34 (1984b)
	Gas work	Lung, bladder, scrotum	Coal carbonization products, beta-naphthylamine	34 (1984b)
	Gas retort house work	Bladder	beta-naphthylamine	34 (1984b)
Rubber industry	Rubber manufacture building	Lymphatic and haematopoietic system (leukaemia)	Benzene	29 (1982b)
	Milling, mixing	Bladder	Aromatic amines	1 (1972)
	Synthetic latex production, tyre curing, calender operating, reclaim, cable making	Bladder	Aromatic amines	4 (1974)
Construction industry	Insulating and pipe covering, demolition work	Lung, pleural and peritoneal mesothelioma	Asbestos	14 (1977)
Leather industry	Boot and shoe manufacture, repair	Nose, bone marrow (leukaemia)	Leather dust, benzene	25 (1980b)
Wood pulp and paper industry	Furniture and cabinet making	Nose (adenocarcinoma)	Wood dust	25 (1980b)
Textile industry	Mule-spinning	Skin	Mineral oils (containing various additives and impurities)	33 (1984a)
Other	Roofing, asphalt work	Lung	Polycyclic aromatic hydrocarbons	35 (1985)
	Jute processing	Skin	Mineral oils (containing various additives and impurities)	33 (1984a)
	Chimney sweeping and other exposures to soot	Scrotum	Polycyclic aromatic hydrocarbons	35 (1985)

As early as 1955, asbestos was clearly demonstrated by Doll to cause lung cancer among people occupationally exposed to it (Doll, 1955). Since then, asbestos has also been found to cause pleural and peritoneal mesothelioma, probably oesophageal, gastric and colorectal cancers, and possibly cancers of the buccal cavity, pharynx and larynx. Talc, which is chemically related to asbestos, has also been studied, and significant excesses of lung cancer mortality have been observed among workers exposed to talc containing asbestiform fibres (Kleinfeld *et al.*, 1967, 1974; Brown and Wagoner, 1979; Selevan *et al.*, 1979; Dement *et al.*, 1980; IARC, 1987).

Vinyl chloride, an important plastics monomer, is one of the latest chemicals that has been shown convincingly to cause cancer in humans exposed occupationally (IARC, 1979). Although vinyl chloride was first reported in 1970 to produce tumours in rats (Viola *et al.*, 1971), measures to reduce levels of exposure of workers to this compound were not taken until 1974, following a report of three cases of the rare angiosarcoma of the liver in heavily exposed workers (Creech and Johnson, 1974). Vinyl chloride is also believed to cause cancers of the brain, lung and lympho-haematopoietic tissues (see Vainio and Saracci, 1986).

Many metal compounds, such as arsenic and certain arsenic compounds, and chromium and certain chromium compounds are known to be carcinogenic to humans (see Table 1; IARC, 1987). Several studies have shown that exposure to inorganic arsenic compounds can increase the risk of lung cancer in smelter workers and workers engaged in the production and use of arsenic-containing pesticides (IARC, 1980a). Investigations on populations living near copper smelters and other point-emission sources of arsenic into the air have also revealed moderate increases in lung cancer mortality (Pershagen, 1985). For many years, arsenic exemplified those agents which, although convincingly carcinogenic to humans, had not been demonstrated to be carcinogenic to experimental animals.

Recently, however, pulmonary carcinomas and/or benign tumours have been induced in hamsters after intratracheal instillations of arsenic trioxide (Ishinishi *et al.*, 1983; Pershagen *et al.*, 1984; Pershagen and Björklund, 1985).

The relatively short list of chemicals causally associated with cancer to which humans are exposed occupationally (Table 1) represents only a fraction of the potential use of epidemiology in occupational cancer. Epidemiological methods have also been used to clearly identify several mixtures as carcinogenic, and exposures in a number of industries have been found to be causally associated with increased incidences of cancer (see Table 2), although the methods have been insufficient to define the specific factors responsible.

Exposures in furniture manufacturing in many countries have been shown to be associated with cancers of the nose and nasal cavities and, in particular, nasal adenocarcinomas (IARC, 1980b). The probable causative factor is wood dust; however, the mechanism by which wood dust could induce cancer is not clear, and it would be necessary to have an animal model in order to understand it better and to identify the exact nature of the causative agent – one of the many natural constituents of wood, the physical properties of the dust particles themselves or one of the many chemicals used in finishing the wood. Evidence that many other organic dusts also appear to put workers at risk of nasal cancer favours the hypothesis that the physical properties of the dust particles are responsible (Brinton *et al.*, 1985; Ng, 1986). It is also interesting to note that some wood dusts contain mutagenic components (Mohtashamipur *et al.*, 1986).

Occupational exposures to mixtures of phenoxyacetic acid herbicides and chlorophenols have also been suggested to be carcinogenic (IARC, 1986). Epidemiological studies in Sweden have suggested that workers exposed to these mixtures are at excess risk for soft tissue sarcomas, Hodgkin's disease and non-Hodgkin's lymphoma (Hardell and Sandström, 1979; Eriksson *et al.*, 1981; Hardell *et al.*, 1981). Although a recent report from Kansas, USA (Hoar *et al.*, 1986) confirmed that non-Hodgkin's lymphoma is associated with the use of herbicides, no increased risk was found for soft tissue sarcoma or for Hodgkin's lymphoma. Studies of similar exposures in New Zealand have also been unable to detect any increased risk of soft tissue sarcomas among pesticides applicators (Smith *et al.*, 1982, 1984).

Workers in the rubber industry are exposed to a large number of agents, and certain occupational exposures in this industry are known to entail increased risks of cancers at multiple sites (IARC, 1982). The increased incidence of bladder cancer was associated with the use of chemicals containing beta-naphthylamine, and the subsequent elimination of this compound resulted in a considerable reduction in bladder cancer risk. A number of recent reports, however, indicate excess mortality from lung and stomach cancer in some sectors of the rubber industry. Lung cancer excesses have been found mainly in occupational groups that are exposed to curing fumes or to industrial solvents, whereas excesses of stomach cancer are associated with occupations involving handling and mixing of raw materials (Nutt, 1983). Although the possible causative factors have not yet been identified, volatile N-nitrosamines have been detected in rubber factories (Spiegelhalder and Preussmann, 1983).

Occupational epidemiology has been fundamental in indicating cancer hazards in the past. By the 1950s, a great diversity of carcinogenic occupational factors, both chemical and physical, had been identified. More recently, occupational cancer epidemiology has been used successfully to identify both very rare types of tumours (such as liver haemangiosarcomas induced by vinyl chloride) and very common types of cancer (such as lung cancer induced by bis(chloromethyl)ether) caused by occupational agents. However, these successes should not conceal the fact that, to date, our ignorance still surpasses our knowledge. More studies, both epidemiological and experimental, are needed to understand the real importance of occupational factors in cancer causation.

From hazard identification to prevention of occupational cancers

Potential and actual carcinogenic risks in the workplace can be identified, and thus reduction of the frequency of human cancers caused by occupational exposure is a practicable objective.

In the case of new chemicals that have not yet been introduced into the workplace, but which have been shown in long-term bioassays to be carcinogenic, risk assessment must be undertaken to determine whether their introduction, and the concomitant safety measures that must be taken to minimize worker exposure, are counterbalanced or outweighed by the benefit that the eventual product will have for the general population. During the introduction of a new chemical, the design of protection for workers can be integrated into the overall process design and should present little additional cost.

Demonstration of the carcinogenic risk, by either experimental or epidemiological studies, of an exposure that already exists may present much greater problems. Re-designing workplaces to install ventilating systems or hoods, introducing automated systems to replace manual operations, and imposing personal hygiene measures or protective clothing and equipment on workers who have long-established habits imply increased costs and much effort in re-training. However, they are essential. It must be accepted that, when cancer researchers have been able to identify a carcinogen in a workplace, no expense or amount of time is too great to prevent worker exposure.

There has been much discussion about the existence of threshold levels for carcinogens (see e.g. Office of Science and Technology Policy, 1985). However, in most countries, the practical approach has been taken which specifies that, even if there is no level below which a carcinogenic effect would not occur, it is necessary to set a limit (e.g. Vainio and Tomatis, 1986). Regulatory policy must, in the first instance, seek to accommodate disparate demands: economic welfare, technological innovation, a clean and safe environment and enhanced quality of life. In order to be able to set such permissible limits of exposure for new and existing chemicals, regulatory bodies rely on research. Such selection requires a combination of epidemiological and laboratory studies, when both are available, or reliance on the results of experimental tests when epidemiological data are not available.

Research in the area of occupational carcinogenesis is guided not only by scientific tradition, but also by considerations arising from the regulatory process. Thus, a number of areas of cancer research, such as the study of DNA-adduct formation and DNA repair, are of additional interest to scientists because they have a bearing on questions (raised by policy-makers) of dosimetry and the existence of a threshold for exposure to carcinogens.

Identification of carcinogenic risks is the most important aspect of preventing occupational cancer; but it is also essential that workers and their environments continue to be monitored, to ensure that control measures to protect workers are effective. Since predictive testing has still not been used sufficiently to ensure that all potential occupational carcinogens have been identified, epidemiological monitoring should be used to detect an unusual occurrence or increased frequency of disease and to relate it to exposure to a previously unsuspected chemical. Only epidemiological studies can provide absolute proof that there is a causal relationship between an exposure and the occurrence of cancer in humans. Although the epidemiological approach is of no help in preventing exposure to 'new' risk factors, it is of prime importance in the surveillance of actions taken and in ensuring that no other risk factors are present in the workplace.

The endpoint of most of the short-term tests used in screening for possible risk is genotoxicity; they are therefore unable to identify factors that act at stages that occur after initiation in the multistage process of carcinogenesis. Epidemiological studies use the 'black box' approach, in which the mechanisms by which cancer is produced are irrelevant. The stage at which a carcinogenic agent is active may, however, be of great importance with respect to intervention measures to reduce the exposure. For instance, agents that act at a later stage (e.g. promoters, antagonist of immunosurveillance) engender a much more rapid response to both the beginning and cessation of exposure than those that act at an early stage (Day, 1985).

Ideally, the purpose of primary prevention of cancer is to detect the environmental risk factors involved in each stage of carcinogenesis and to eliminate them. In reality, existing short-term tests detect many factors involved at the initiation stage but not those involved in later stages of carcinogenesis. Results from laboratory and epidemiological studies strongly suggest that elimination not only of initiating agents but also of those involved in tumour promotion would be an effective means of cancer prevention.

Occupational cancer provides an excellent ground for primary prevention. Constant improvements in methods of environmental and biological monitoring allow the identification of exposures with progressively greater precision. Increased awareness of occupational health problems has improved the accuracy of record keeping, and thus, together with the possibility of prior identification of carcinogenic risks on the basis of experimental data, the health of workers can be protected by efficient epidemiological surveillance.

Conclusion

Reduction to an insignificant level of the frequency of human cancer caused by occupational exposures is a practicable and attainable objective. At present, selective reduction of the most significant exposures is the most realistic goal and the only practical means of progress; thus, the first requirement is to identify and reduce the significant sources of exposures. Such selection of targets will require a combination of epidemiological and laboratory studies. At the same time, predictive testing must be used to minimize the introduction of additional carcinogens into the workplace.

Monitoring of the environment and the human population must be continued to ensure that controls are effective and that cancer risk in workers is reduced. Predictive testing cannot identify all potential human carcinogens and, thus, epidemiological monitoring for the unusual occurrence or increased frequency of common cancers is important.

References

Brinton, L.A., Blot, W.J. and Frauemeni, J. (1985) Nasal cancer in the textile and clothing industries, *Br. J. Ind. Med.* **42**, 469–474.

Brown, D.P. and Wagoner, J.K. (1979) Mortality patterns among miners and millers occupationally exposed to asbestiform talc. In Dement, J.M. and Lemen, R. (eds.) *Dusts and disease*, Panthotox Publishers, Park Forst South, 317–324.

Cook, J.W., Hieger, I., Kennaway, E.L. and Mayneord, W.V. (1932) The production of cancer by pure hydrocarbons. Part I, *Proc. R. Soc. London Ser. B III:* 455–484.

Creech, J.L. Jr, Johnson, M.N. (1974) Angiosarcoma of liver in the manufacture of polyvinyl chloride, *J. Occup. Med.* **16**, 150–151.

Day, N.E. (1985) Risk estimation models. In Vouck, V.B., Butler, G.C., Hoel, D.G. and Peakall, D.B. (eds.) *Methods for estimating risk of chemical injury: human and non-human biota and ecosystems*, John Wiley & Sons, New York, 381–393.

Dement, J.M., Zumwalde, R.D., Gamble, J.F., Fellner, W., De Meo, M.J., Brown, D.P. and Wagner, J.K. (1980) *Occupational exposure to talc containing asbestos.* NIOSH technical report series, DHEW (NIOSH) publication no. 80–115. National Institute for Occupational Safety and Health, Cincinnati, OH.

Doll, R. (1955) Mortality from lung cancer in asbestos workers, *Br. J. Ind. Med.* **12**, 81–86.

Eriksson, M., Hardell, L., Berg, N.O., Moller, T. and Axelson, O. (1981) Soft-tissue sarcomas and exposure to chemical substances: a case referent study, *Br. J. Ind. Med.* **38**, 27–33.

Hardell, L. and Sandström, A. (1979) Case-control study: soft-tissue sarcomas and exposure to phenoxyacetic acids or chlorophenols, *Br. J. Cancer* **39**, 11–17.

Hardell, L., Eriksson, M., Lenner, P. and Lundgren, E. (1981) Malignant lymphoma and exposure to chemicals, especially organic solvents, chlorophenols and phenoxy acids: a case control study, *Br. J. Cancer* **43**, 169–176.

Hoar, S.K., Blair, A., Holmes, F.F., Boysen, C.D., Robel, R.J., Hoover, R. and Fraumeni, J.F. (1986) Agricultural herbicide use and risk of lymphoma and soft-tissue sarcoma, *J. Am. Med. Assoc.* **256**, 1141–1147.

Hueper, W.C., Wiley, F.H. and Wolfe, H.D. (1938) Experimental production of bladder tumours in dogs by administration of beta-naphthylamine, *J. Ind. Hyg. Toxicol.* **20**, 46–48.

IARC (1972) IARC monographs on the evaluation of carcinogenic risk of chemicals to man, vol. 1, *Some inorganic substances, chlorinated hydrocarbons, aromatic amines, N-nitroso compounds and natural products.* International Agency for Research on Cancer, Lyon.

IARC (1974) IARC monographs on the evaluation of carcinogenic risk of chemicals to man, vol. 4, *Some aromatic amines, hydrazine and related substances, N-nitroso compounds and miscellaneous aklylating agents*. International Agency for Research on Cancer, Lyon.

IARC (1976) IARC monographs on the evaluation of carcinogenic risk of chemicals to man, vol 11, Cadmium, nickel, some epoxides, miscellaneous industrial chemicals and general considerations on volatile anaesthetics. International Agency for Research on Cancer, Lyon.

IARC (1977) IARC monographs on the evaluation of carcinogenic risk of chemicals to man, vol. 14, *Asbestos*. International Agency for Research on Cancer, Lyon.

IARC (1979) IARC monographs on the evaluation of the carcinogenic risk of chemicals to humans, vol. 19, *Some monomers, plastics and synthetic elastomers, and acrolein*. International Agency for Research on Cancer, Lyon.

IARC (1980a) IARC monographs on the evaluation of the carcinogenic risk of chemicals to humans, vol. 23, *Some metals and metallic compounds*. International Agency for Research on Cancer, Lyon.

IARC (1980b) IARC monographs on the evaluation of the carcinogenic risk of chemicals to humans, vol. 25, *Wood, leather, and some associated industries*. International Agency for Research on Cancer, Lyon.

IARC (1982) IARC monographs on the evaluation of the carcinogenic risk of chemicals to humans, vol. 28, *The rubber industry*, International Agency for Research on Cancer, Lyon.

IARC (1982) IARC monographs on the evaluation of the carcinogenic risk of chemicals to humans, vol. 29, *Some industrial chemicals and dyestuffs*. International Agency for Research on Cancer, Lyon.

IARC (1983) *Approaches to classifying chemical carcinogens according to mechanism of action* (IARC internal technical report no. 83/001). International Agency for Research on Cancer, Lyon.

IARC (1984a) IARC monographs on the evaluation of the carcinogenic risk of chemicals to humans, vol. 33, *Polynuclear aromatic compounds, part 2, carbon blacks, mineral oils and some nitroarenes*. International Agency for Research on Cancer, Lyon.

IARC (1984b) IARC monographs on the evaluation of the carcinogenic risk of chemicals to humans, vol. 34, *Polynuclear aromatic compounds, part 3, industrial exposures in aluminium production, coal gasification, coke production, and iron and steel founding*. International Agency for Research on Cancer, Lyon.

IARC (1985) IARC monographs on the evaluation of the carcinogenic risk of chemicals to humans, vol. 35, *Polynuclear aromatic compounds, part 4, bitumens, coal-tars and derived products, shale-oils and soots*. International Agency for Research on Cancer, Lyon.

IARC (1986) IARC monographs on the evaluation of the carcinogenic risk of chemicals to humans, vol. 41, *Some halogenated hydrocarbons and pesticide exposures*. International Agency for Research on Cancer, Lyon.

IARC (1987) IARC monographs on the evaluation of the carcinogenic risk of chemicals to humans, suppl. 7, *Chemicals, occupational exposures and cultural habits associated with cancer in humans, vols. 1–42*. International Agency for Research on Cancer, Lyon.

International Labour Office (1921) *Cancer of the bladder among workers in aniline factories*. Studies and reports series no. 1., Geneva, pp1–26.

Ishinishi, I., Yamamoto, A., Hisanaga, A. and Inamasu, T. (1983) Tumorigenicity of arsenic trioxide to the lung in Syrian golden hamsters by intermittent instillations, *Cancer Lett.* **21**, 141–147.

Kleinfeld, M., Messite, J., Kooyman, O. and Zaki, M.H. (1967) Mortality among talc miners and millers in New York state, *Arch. Environ. Health* **14**, 663–667.

MacLure, K.M. and MacMahon, B. (1980) An epidemiologic perspective of environmental carcinogenesis, *Epidemiol. Rev.* **2**, 19–48.

Merletti, F., Heseltine, E., Saracci, R., Simonato, L., Vainio, H. and Wilbourn, J. (1984) Target organs for carcinogenicity of chemicals and industrial exposures in humans, *Cancer Res.* **44**, 2244–2250.

Mohtashamipur, E., Norpoth, K. and Hallerberg, B. (1986) A fraction of beech wood mutagenic in the Salmonella/mammalian microsome assay, *Int. Arch. Occup. Environ. Health* **58**, 227–234.

Ng, T.P. (1986) A case-referent study of cancer of the nasal cavity and sinuses in Hong Kong, *Int. J. Epidemiol.* **15**, 171–175.

Nutt, A. (1983) Rubber work and health – past, present and perspective, *Scand. J. Work Environ. Health* **9**, (Suppl. 2) 49–57.

Office of Science and Technology Policy (1985) *Chemical carcinogens : a review of the science and its associated principles*, Fed. Reg., March **14**, 10371–10442.

Pershagen, G. (1985) Lung cancer mortality among men living near an arsenic emitting smelter, *Am. J. Epidemiol.* **122**, 684–694.

Pershagen, G. and Björkland, N.E. (1985) On the pulmonary tumorigenicity of arsenic trisulfide and calcium arsenate in hamsters, *Cancer Lett.* **27**, 99–104.

Pershagen, G., Nordberg, G. and Björkland, N.E. (1984) Carcinomas of the respiratory tract in hamsters given arsenic trioxide and/or benzo(a)pyrene by the pulmonary route, *Environ. Res.* **34**, 227–241.

Pott, P. (1775) *Chirurgical observations relative to the cataract, the polypus of the nose, the cancer of the scrotum, the different kinds of ruptures and the mortification of the toes and feet*, Hawes, Clarke and Collins, London, 63–65.

Rehn, L. (1895) Blasengeschwülste bei Fuchsin-Arbeitern, *Arch. klin. Chir.* **50**, 588–600.

Schmähl, D. and Kaldor, J. (eds.) (1986) *Carcinogenicity of alkylating cytostatic drugs*. IARC scientific publications, vol 78. International Agency for Research on Cancer, Lyon.

Selevan, S.G., Dement, J.M., Wagoner, J.K. and Froines, J.R. (1979) Mortality patterns among miners and millers of non-asbestiform talc: preliminary report. In Lemen, R. and Dement, J.M. (eds.) *Dusts and disease*, Pathotox Publishers, Park Forest South, IL, 379–388.

Smith, A.H., Fisher, D.O., Pearce, N.E. and Teague, C.A. (1982) Do agricultural chemicals cause soft tissue sarcoma? Initial findings of a case-control study in New Zealand, *Community Health Stud.* **6**, 114–119.

Smith, A.H., Pearce, N.E., Fisher, D.O., Giles, H.J. Teague, C.A. and Howard, J.K. (1984) Soft tissue sarcoma and exposure to phenoxyherbicides and chlorophenols in New Zealand, *J. Natl. Cancer Inst.* **73**, 1111–1117.

Sorsa, M., Hemminki, K. and Vainio, H. (1985) Occupational exposure to anticancer drugs – potential and real hazards, *Mutat. Res.* **154**, 135–149.

Spiegelhalder, B. and Preussmann, R. (1983) Occupational nitrosamine exposure. 1. Rubber and type industry, *Carcinogenesis* **4**, 1137–1152.

Vainio, H. and Saracci, R. (1986) Carcinogenicity of selected vinyl compounds, some aldehydes, haloethyl nitrosoureas and furocoumarins: an overview. In Singer, B. and Bartsch, H. (eds.) *The role of cyclic nucleic acid adducts in carcinogenesis and mutagenesis*, IARC scientific publications, vol 70. International Agency for Research on Cancer, Lyon, 15–29.

Vainio, H. and Tomatis, L. (1986) Exposure to carcinogens: an overview of scientific and regulatory aspects, *Appl. Ind. Hyg.* **1**, 42–48.

Vainio, H., Hemminki, K. and Wilbourn, J. (1985) Data on the carcinogenicity of chemicals in the IARC Monographs programme, *Carcinogenesis* **6**, 1653–1665.

Viola, P.L., Bigotti, A. and Caputo, A. (1971) Oncogenic response of rat skin, lungs and bones to vinyl chloride, *Cancer Res.* **31**, 516–522.

LOW LEVEL RADIATION AND THE PREVENTION OF CANCERS

Roger Milne

Introduction

Radiation is a fact of life. Light and heat from the sun are natural forms of it that are essential to human existence. Certain human activities also generate forms of radiation: microwaves for cooking, radiowaves for communication, radar for navigation and x-rays for medical investigations.

Emissions from radioactive substances are a further source of radiation. Some of these substances occur naturally throughout the environment, others are human productions.

There are two classes of radiation – ionizing and non-ionizing. The former produces an electrical effect called ionization when it strikes matter.

Ionizing radiation includes cosmic rays, x-rays and the radiations emitted by the radioactive decay of radioactive substances. One such source is the nuclear power and weapons industries which make extensive use of radioactive substances. In the non-ionizing category are heat, light, radar, radiowaves and microwaves.

The most worrying effect of ionizing radiation is the fact that exposed people can develop malignant diseases – specifically cancers – as well as inherited effects in their descendants. The likelihood of radiation-induced effects is related to the dose of radiation received, irrespective of whether the radiation is of natural or artificial origin (BEIR, 1980).

In the case of non-ionizing radiation, effects are dependent on the specific type and intensity of the radiation. They include damage to the skin and eye and, for those radiations that penetrate body tissues, damage to internal organs due to excessive heating. In the long term, skin cancer and cataracts may result from exposure to some forms of non-ionizing radiation.

There are also different types of ionizing radiations. The three main types are called alpha, beta and gamma. Each has a different penetrating power. Alpha radiation is easily stopped by a piece of paper or card. Alpha emitters can only be dangerous if they are swallowed or breathed into the body. Beta radiation can be stopped by a sheet of metal foil. And gamma radiation needs a thick wall of concrete, lead or steel to stop it.

Scientists use special units to quantify radiation and to measure its effect on people. The basic unit is the millisievert (mSv). On average we are exposed to a total of about 1 mSv of radiation each year, directly from outer space, and from naturally radioactive materials in the ground, in the walls of buildings and in our own bodies. The becquerel (Bq) is the unit used to measure radioactivity. It is a measure of the rate at which the unstable nuclei change. The gray (Gy) is the unit used to describe the quantity of energy imparted by ionizing radiation to unit mass of matter such as tissue.

If the whole body is exposed to a very high dose of radiation, death may occur within a matter of weeks: an instantaneous absorbed dose of about 5 Gy or more would probably be lethal, provided that no treatment was given, as a result of damage to the bone marrow and gastrointestinal tract.

The most important late effect of radiation is cancer. The fundamental processes by which cancer is induced by radiation are not fully understood, but a greater incidence of various malignant diseases have been observed in groups of people who were exposed to high doses of radiation years previously. Each exposed person has an extra chance of contracting a cancer that depends largely on the dose received. The situation is analogous to smoking, where those who smoke most run the highest risk of lung cancer, but by no means all of them will contract it. There is no way at present of distinguishing cancers caused by radiation from those that occur for other reasons.

Establishing risk factors for cancer caused by radiation is essentially a mathematical exercise. If the number of people in an irradiated group and the doses that they have received are known, and if the number of cancers eventually observed in the group exceeds the number that would be expected in an otherwise similar but non-irradiated group, the excess number of cancers may be attributed to radiation, and the risk of cancer per unit dose equivalent calculated.

The main source of information on the risk of radiation-induced cancer following exposure to whole-body gamma radiation comes from follow-up studies on the survivors of the atomic bombs dropped on Hiroshima and Nagasaki (Preston and Pierce, 1987). Risk estimates for x-radiation and gamma radiation can also be obtained for a number of tissues from human populations treated with external radiation for non-malignant conditions or for diagnostic purposes and from people exposed to nuclear weapons fallout in the Pacific. Data on the effects of alpha emitters come from miners exposed to the naturally-produced radioactive gas radon, from workers exposed to radium in the luminizing industry, from patients given radium-224 for the treatment of disease and from patients given the x-ray contrast medium Thorotrast (thorium oxide).

Cancer risks derived from the Japanese populations and other exposed groups are based largely on exposures at high dose delivered over a short period of time. In practice most people are exposed to low levels of radiation over long time periods. It is generally assumed that there is a simple proportional relationship between dose and risk, although there is some evidence that the picture is different depending on the type of radiation involved. For beta, gamma and x radiation the risks seems to be less at low doses and low dose rates. At present, there is no sound basis for assuming that there is any threshold below which cancers and hereditary defects do not occur.

The latest internationally accepted radiological protection guidelines, formulated by the International Commission on Radiological Protection (ICRP), assume that the risk factor is now between three and five times greater than once believed (ICRP, 1991).

Currently someone living in the UK has an average annual effective radiation dose of around 2.5 mSv. Natural background radiation accounts for 1 mSv and about the same amount again is produced by radon gas in buildings. Medical sources, fall out from testing nuclear weapons, occupational exposure and radioactive discharges from nuclear sites make up the remainder.

According to Britain's National Radiological Protection Board (NRPB), the small number of people (known as the 'critical group') exposed to the highest levels of radioactivity from discharges from nuclear industry sites had, in the late 1980s, a 1 in 70,000 risk of contracting a fatal cancer (NRPB, 1989). This contrasts with a 1 in 200 risk of fatal lung cancer faced by a smoker using 10 cigarettes a day. At the same time the annual risk of death in a UK road accident is about 1 in 9,500. On the present risk factors, if an individual was exposed to 1,000 mSv the risk of cancer would increase from 25 per cent to 27 per cent. This is an average figure for men and women, old and young. In fact the risk of radiation to women is slightly higher than that of men because of the possibility of breast cancer, and children may be about twice as vulnerable as adults to radiation. Babies in the womb are more vulnerable still.

Radon

As many as 2,500 deaths every year in Britain due to lung cancer could be the result of exposure to radon.

Radon is a radioactive gas formed in the earth from the decay of uranium. All earth and masonry materials contain small quantities of uranium. Radon, then, is continuously created under buildings and trapped within them.

In homes in the UK the concentration of radon is on average 20 Bq per cubic metre of air (20 Bq m^3). In some parts of the country relatively large numbers of houses have very high concentrations of radon. The highest recorded in Britain is over 8,000 Bq m^3 (NRPB, 1987a).

In 1987, the NRPB, concerned that the risk posed by exposure to radon was not being taken seriously enough, formally advised that concentrations of the gas in homes should be drastically reduced (NRPB, 1987b). It recommended that an action level of 200 Bq m^3 should be accepted as the basis for remedial work. According to recent preliminary survey work, as many as 100,000 British homes may exceed that action level. The final tally could be as high as 230,000. Most are in hard rock areas of the country like Cornwall, Devon, Somerset, Northamptonshire and north east Scotland.

Indoor radon levels high enough to cause concern are almost always due to radon from the underlying soil and/or rock. The air pressure indoors is often slightly lower than that in the soil, and air from the soil containing radon tends to be drawn from the ground into the house via small cracks and service entry points.

Limiting radon entry, rather than removing indoor radon, is the preferred remedy. A two-stage process is recommended by the government on the advice of its Building Research Establishment. Firstly, ground-level floors should be sealed (i.e. by using polythene sheet). Secondly, the underfloor pressure should be reduced. For suspended floors this is achieved by increasing the ventilation under the floor; for solid floors the approach is to create a small sump under the house from which the radon-laden air can be drawn out through a pipe by a fan.

The extent and nature of the health effects of radon gas are the subject of some controversy. Some scientists question whether radon does cause cancer on the scale suggested by NRPB. On the other hand, some recent research suggests there may be an association between exposure to radon and a number of other cancers, previously unsuspected of being linked with radon.

The NRPB calculations of risk have all been extrapolated from data on miners. To date no British epidemiological studies have been completed on exposure to actual doses in the home. Studies are underway but the results won't be known for some years yet.

The British Department of Health, for instance, suggests that the NRPB risk factors may be skewed because the epidemiological studies of miners were based on high levels of radon (Department of Health, 1991). The miners, it is also suggested, may have been exposed to rock dusts containing other radioactive material or to other toxic substances.

Two British research groups have recently published papers on other possible cancer risks associated with domestic exposure to radon. Both are highly speculative. Dr. Henshaw of Bristol University claims that the dose received by different organs exposed to radon is higher than previously thought and claims to have found possible geographical correlations between radon exposure and a number of other cancers, including myeloid leukaemia, melanoma and prostate cancer (Henshaw, 1991).

In addition, the Leukaemia Research Fund Epidemiology Research Unit has produced an atlas of leukaemia incidence which suggests a correlation of acute lymphoblastic leukaemia in children in areas of England with high levels of radon (Cartwright, 1991). If these studies are confirmed, radon could be more hazardous than the NRPB currently assumes. Dr. Henshaw, for instance, suggests that as many as 4,500 deaths a year could be attributed to radon, nearly double the NRPB estimate (Henshaw, 1991).

Nuclear energy

There has been considerable speculation in the UK that nuclear installations may be responsible for clusters of childhood cancers known by the generic name leukaemia. There are several different types of leukaemia, and of the closely related diseases, lymphoma.

Leukaemia is relatively rare, affecting about 1 in 1,800 live births or about 500 children per year in the UK. It kills more children between the ages of 2 and 15 than any other disease, but recent improvements in treatment mean that nowadays the cure rate for children is better than 60 per cent.

Leukaemia can start with damage to the DNA of a single primitive blood cell in the bone marrow. Several agents are known to cause damage to DNA, such as ionizing radiation, ultraviolet light, chemicals such as benzene, and some viruses. Genetic factors may also play a part. Also implicated are certain chemotherapeutic drugs, maternal smoking during pregnancy and garden pesticides.

Eight years ago a TV programme, investigating the Sellafield nuclear complex, uncovered an excessive number of cases of juvenile leukaemia in Seascale, 3 miles south of Sellafield on the North West coast of England in Cumbria. According to this programme, there had been seven cases when on average less than one would have been expected.

A government-appointed committee of inquiry was set up to consider the programme's findings. The inquiry confirmed that there was an excess of leukaemia in the area but said more research was needed to confirm – or deny – a causal link with

radiation from the Sellafield site (Black, 1984). Subsequently the government set up a further body, the Committee on the Medical Aspects of Radiation in the Environment (COMARE) to keep a watching brief on the subject.

In the last few years there have been a plethora of studies investigating cancer rates near nuclear sites.

COMARE reassessed the Seascale and Sellafield information, confirmed an excess of childhood leukaemias, but said it was difficult to explain in terms of radioactive discharges (COMARE, 1986). Another COMARE report looked at a leukaemia cluster around the Dounreay nuclear research establishment in northern Scotland, home of Britain's fast reactor programme (COMARE, 1988). Dounreay also has a reprocessing plant, though much smaller than the one at Sellafield. A significant excess leukaemia rate was confirmed but the committee could not find a definite causal link with radiation from the site. A third COMARE investigation found a small but significant excess of childhood cancers in the population around the military nuclear weapons sites of Aldermaston and Burghfield (COMARE, 1989).

Meanwhile, a large-scale and definitive study carried out by the Office of Population Censuses and Surveys (OPCS) established that overall cancer rates around civic nuclear power stations were, save for some exceptions, below average (Cook-Mozaffari *et al.*, 1987). Studies in France and the US have been equally inconclusive.

Scientists are currently unable to explain why the excesses identified around some nuclear sites have occurred. The excesses near Sellafield, Dounreay, Aldermaston and Burghfield all involve about 5 to 15 cases. Yet Sellafield's discharges of radioactive pollution are about 15 times greater than Dounreay's which are in turn about 900 times greater than those from Aldermaston and Burghfield. The effect seems to be independent of the amount and type of radioactive material released by the site under scrutiny.

Other causes than ionizing radiation have been suggested. These range from other chemicals, a rare radioactive substance, a combination of those factors and even a viral source. To date the evidence is very inconclusive and highly speculative.

In 1990, a study showed a link between paternal occupation and leukaemia (Gardner *et al.*, 1990). Men working in the nuclear reprocessing industry in Cumbria ran a raised risk of fathering children who developed leukaemia. The fathers of four of the five leukaemic cases born in Seascale are known to have worked at Sellafield and have received cumulative doses of at least 97 mSv prior to conception. This link between paternal radiation and subsequent juvenile leukaemia was entirely unexpected. The atomic bomb survivor studies have not demonstrated a similar possible link. A similar reappraisal of the Dounreay data (Urquhart *et al.*, 1991) neither proved nor disproved the link between parental occupation and the development of leukaemia.

The 1990 Gardner report does seem to suggest that people living near Sellafield but without direct connection with the plant are at no risk: if paternal exposure to radiation is the cause, perhaps via a chromosomal alteration, discharges from the plant are unlikely to be relevant. The arguments will continue for some time to come[15].

What they have done is reinforce the need to keep worker exposure to all forms of radiations as low as possible as a prudent precautionary measure.

Conclusions

Current scientific evidence suggests that low-level radiation poses a small risk of causing cancers. However, it has been pointed out recently that the risk of fatal cancer is a poor measure of the consequences of exposures to ionizing radiation. Should we adopt a more sophisticated approach to take account of the time and nature of death in addition to its probability?

One possibility is to look at the 'number of years lost' rather than the number of deaths. On this basis the difference between the predictions of the relative and absolute risk models is not as pronounced. Is a slow death from cancer more acceptable than a sudden death from a road accident? Do we find a plane crash more acceptable if the passengers are old age pensioners? 'These are problems for moral philosophy, not for science, and they need to be seriously addressed'[17].

While the arguments continue, the imperatives for radiological protection remain. Exposure of public and workers to ionizing radiation must be kept as low as possible.

In the case of non-ionizing radiation there is no doubt that the biggest risk posed is skin cancer from exposure to ultraviolet radiation.

Cutaneous malignant melanoma, while much less frequently occurring than the common non-melanoma skin cancers, is much more serious and accounts for the majority of deaths from skin cancer. The trend of increased incidence of malignant melanoma in developed countries is a cause for concern for public health and particularly among susceptible white populations living in tropical and sub-tropical latitudes.

A scientific debate has begun over the health implications of electrical and magnetic fields, both of which are further categories of non-ionizing radiation. To date the epidemiological evidence of diverse health effects – birth defects and a variety of cancers – is equivocal.

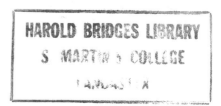
HAROLD BRIDGES LIBRARY
S MARTIN'S COLLEGE
LANCASTER

References

BEIR III Committee on the Biological Effects of Ionizing Radiation (1980) *The effects on population of exposure to low levels of ionizing radiations*, National Academy of Sciences, National Academy Press, Washington.

Black, Sir D. *et al.* (1986) *Investigation of the possible increased incidence of cancers in West Cumbria: report of the Independent Advisory Group*, HMSO (1984).

COMARE (1986) First Report, HMSO.

COMARE (1988) Second Report, HMSO.

COMARE (1989) Third Report, HMSO.

Cook-Mozaffari, P.J. *et al.* (1987) *Cancer incidence and mortality in the vicinity of nuclear installations, England and Wales 1959–80*. OPCS, HMSO .

Cartwright, Dr., Director of the Leukaemia Research Centre. Memorandum to the House of Commons Select Committee on the Environment. ibid.

Department of Health memorandum (1991) *Evidence to the House of Commons Select Committee on the Environment session 1990-1991*. Published in Sixth Report Indoor Pollution Minutes of Evidence (volume 11), HMSO.

Gardner, M.J. *et al.* (1990) Results of a case control study of leukaemia and lymphoma among young poeple near Sellafield nuclear plant in West Cumbria, *Brit. Med. J.* **300**, 423–429.

Henshaw, Dr. (1986) Oral evidence to the House of Commons Select Committee on the Environment (1991).

International Commission on Radiological Protection (1991) *Recommendations of the ICRP*, ICRP Publications 60. *Annals of the ICRP* **21** (1–3).

National Radiological Protection Board (1987a) *Exposure to radon daughters in dwellings*. Report NRPB-G56, HMSO.

National Radiological Protection Board (1987b) press statement, January.

National Radiological Protection Board (1989) *Living with Radiation*, fourth edition, HMSO.

Preston, D.L. and Pierce, D.A. (1987) *The effects of changes in dosimetry on cancer mortality risk estimates in the atom bomb survivors*. RERF-TR9-87. Hiroshima Effects Research Foundation.

Sumner, D.(1990) *Medicine and war* **6**, 112–19.

Urquhart, J. *et al.* (1991) Case control study of leukaemia and non-Hodgkins lymphoma in children in Caithness around the Dounreay nuclear installation, *MBJ*, **302**, 687–692.

STRESS AND PSYCHOLOGICAL ASPECTS OF CANCERS

Steven Greer

Introduction

The notion that stressful life experiences and personality attributes may contribute to the causes of cancer is not new. In the second century, the famous physician Galen claimed that cancer occurred more commonly in 'melancholic' women than in those of 'sanguine temperament' (Mettler and Mettler, 1947). Various physicians and surgeons in the 18th and 19th centuries reported case histories which suggested a possible link between psychological factors and the subsequent appearance of cancer. The state of the art was summarized in 1846 in a review by Walshe (1846):

> Much has been written on the influence of mental misery, sudden reverses of fortune, and habitual gloominess of temper on the desposition of carcinomatous matter ... whether this be the real catenation of circumstances or not, and although the alleged influence of mental disquietude has never been made a matter of demonstration it would be vain to deny that facts of a very convincing character in respect to the agency of the mind in production of this disease are frequently observed.

One hundred and fifty years later, Walshe's comments remain relevant. There is still no absolute, conclusive proof of a link between stress and personality attributes on the one hand and cancer on the other.

This is hardly surprising, given the inherent complexity of the topic and the daunting problems faced by researchers in this field (Greer and Morris, 1978). For example, we do not know with any degree of accuracy when cancers start. By the time the disease manifests itself clinically, several years have usually elapsed since its onset. Hence, we cannot be certain whether any stressful event preceded the actual onset of cancer. Moreover, the longer a person is asked to remember, the greater the likelihood of faulty recall. The cancer diagnosis itself may also influence recall of stressful events; some patients try to find a reason for the inexplicable development of cancer in past life experiences. The actual measurement of stress is also problematic. Measures range from life event questionnaires which list a series of arbitrarily weighted events irrespective of their impact on the person, to clinical interviews which rely entirely on subjective events. Some of these difficulties also apply to the assessment of personality traits.

These comments do not imply that such methodological problems are insurmountable, or that research in this area is fruitless. But we need to be aware of the difficulties involved in investigating a possible link between psychological factors and cancer. Opinions on this hypothesis should be based on a dispassionate appraisal of available scientific evidence. Several scientifically rigorous studies have been reported. The evidence emerging from these studies is considered below.

First, however, we shall examine the concept of stress and attempt to show how – theoretically – stress and other psychological factors could contribute to the development and progress of cancer.

The concept of stress

Stress is a vague term often misused by the media to explain many human ills. Even in the scientific literature, there is no generally agreed definition of stress. The term is variously used to describe:

(a) an environmental stimulus to which the individual (i.e. human or other animal) has to adapt;

(b) the way in which such a stimulus is perceived;

(c) the psychological and/or physiological responses to the stimulus;

(d) the interaction between environmental stimuli and the individual's adaptive (coping) responses.

Many studies by psychiatrists and behavioural scientists have explored the links between psychological stressors and subsequent psychopathological responses, such as anxiety states and depressive reactions. Parallel studies have focussed on psychobiological relationships, i.e. the effect of psychological stressors on bodily processes and, consequently, on the development of disease.

Psychological stressors, in the present context, refer to those adverse life experiences which result in severe sustained emotional disturbance. It is important to note that stressors cannot be defined independently of the person and his or her circumstances. For example, the death of a pet will probably have no discernible effect on an adult leading a full life at home and work. But the same event may well produce severe emotional distress in an elderly person who is friendless and living alone. Another important factor which should be taken into account is the person's coping ability. This can greatly modify the severity and duration of stressor-induced emotional disturbance.

A psychobiological model of cancer

Clearly, the hypothesis that adverse life experiences are a direct cause of any disease – let alone cancers – is simplistic and untenable. The theoretical model of stressor-induced disease illustrated in Figure 1 is more in line with the current state of knowledge.

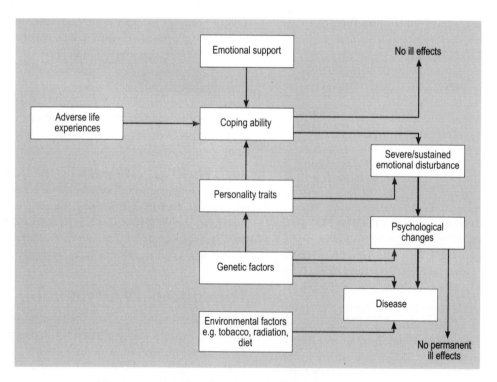

Figure 1   Theoretical model of stressor-induced disease

The question is, do any physiological mechanisms exist through which stress and other psychological factors could influence cancer development? One obvious and direct link between psychological factors and the development of cancer is the individual's behaviour. This, of course, is a function of personality. It has been firmly established that certain behaviours are important causes of several kinds of cancer. Tobacco smoking and excessive alcohol consumption are two well known examples of such carcinogenic behaviour (Doll and Peto, 1982).

Far less is known about physiological mechanisms which supposedly mediate psychological influences in tumour growth. To date, no evidence has been published which identifies the physiological pathway(s) *actually* involved in transmitting psychological influences on tumour growth in humans.

Since no specific intermediary physiological pathways have been identified, the question that arises is which pathways – if any – could, in theory, mediate the effects of psychological stressors on tumour growth. The brief summary presented here is based on a paper by Pettingale (1985).

In general terms, cancer is a disorder of cell growth which involves some imbalance in normal tissue regulation (homeostasis). Many mechanisms contribute to the control of tissue homeostasis, including some which are capable of being influenced by psychological factors. Clearly, psychological factors can only be mediated by the central nervous system. Under certain conditions (see Figure 1), psychological stressors can trigger the release of various so-called 'stress' hormones and neuropeptides through the limbic-hypothalmic-pituitary pathway. The resulting physiological changes produce alterations in many tissues as described by Pettingale (1985). In addition, impairment of the immune system (the body's defence system) may affect tumour growth or spread (Herberman, 1981). The immune system is itself under neuroendocrine control (Besedovski and Sorkin, 1977; Tecoma

and Huey, 1985). The sensitivity of the neuroendocrine system to psychological factors is firmly established (Guillemin *et al.*, 1977; Stein *et al.*, 1985; Pert *et al.*, 1985). Hence, the neuroendocrine system – by its direct effect on tissues and by its control of the immune system – provides the principal pathways through which psychological factors could, in theory, influence the development of tumours. A simplified diagrammatic representation of these pathways is shown in Figure 2. The dotted arrows indicate that the connections between the pathways are bi-directional.

This brief summary does scant justice to the exceedingly complex and incompletely understood interactions between the nervous, endocrine and immune systems and their influence on tumour growth (Greer and Brady, 1988; Irwin and Asisman, 1984; Razavi *et al.*, 1990). The pathways mentioned here are affected by psychological factors but the connection between these factors and tumour growth through these pathways is speculative.

Psychological factors in the development and course of cancer

From the foregoing discussion, we can formulate a broad hypothesis which may be stated as follows.

Whatever the random mutation or other biological initiators of the cancer process, its further development depends in part upon the homeostatic controls which restrain or stimulate all tissue growth. It is postulated that psychological factors influence these homeostatic controls thereby contributing to tumour growth or restraint. This hypothesis does *not* state that psychological factors are necessary or sufficient causes. Rather, it is postulated that, among multiple biological causes of cancer, psychological factors may play a part in (i) predisposing individuals to certain cancers, and (ii) worsening or, conversely, improving outcome.

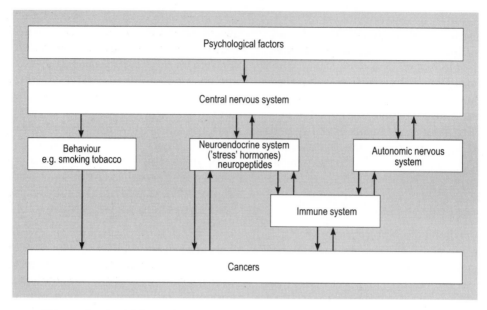

Figure 2 Possible pathways between psychological factors and cancer

Psychological factors contributing to the development of cancer

Psychological stressors

A voluminous literature on animal experiments exists. Animals have been subjected to a variety of psychological and physical stressors to determine their effect on the incidence and growth rate of experimentally induced or transplanted tumours. Sadly, such procedures tell us more about the minds of the researchers than about the postulated stress–cancer link. These experiments are unacceptable on ethical grounds. They are also scientifically dubious. Reported results have been confusing, some suggesting that stress increased tumour incidence and growth, others indicating no effect and yet others suggesting that stress has an inhibitory effect on tumour growth (Burgess, 1978).

Not surprisingly, Peters and Mason (1979) in their review of the literature concluded that 'experimental support can be found for essentially any view concerning the effect of

stress on neoplasia'. Whatever the results of such animal experiments, the extreme stress-inducing procedures used have no relevance to the ordinary stressful situations that are experienced by humans. In investigating the effect of stress on humans, scientists would do well to heed Alexander Pope's dictum: 'The proper study of mankind is man.'

Many clinical observations have suggested the possibility that psychological stressors, such as bereavement, may predispose individuals to develop cancer (Le Shan, 1959). These observations have stimulated a number of systematic, controlled clinical investigations in which patients with cancer are compared with 'control' subjects.

Several controlled studies have failed to demonstrate any significant differences between women with breast cancer and control subjects in incidence of stressful events – including loss of a loved person – during the previous five years (Muslin *et al.*, 1966; Greer and Morris, 1975; Schonfield, 1975) or during childhood (Muslin *et al.*, 1966). The control subjects in these studies were women with benign breast disease. Since a small proportion of patients with benign disease may eventually develop cancer, a more recent study used two control groups, viz. women with benign breast disease and women who had no evidence of any breast disease. The incidence of stressful events in the preceding three years was again similar in the cancer group and the two control groups (Priestman et al., 1985).

Only one control study of women with breast cancer (Cooper et al., 1989) has reported differences between these patients and control subjects who had benign breast disease or were healthy; unusually, some of the control subjects were drawn from a private 'well woman' clinic. An increased incidence of bereavement in the previous two years was reported by cancer patients, but many other stressors were reported less frequently by these patients than by control subjects.

The most interesting result, however, was the strong correlation found between cancer and the perceived impact of the stressor. In other words, the cancer patients rated stressors – particularly death of loved person – as having had a greater impact than was the case among control subjects. This result suggests that women who develop breast cancer may have had greater difficulty in coping with previous psychological stressors than control subjects.

Two controlled studies of patients with lung cancer have yielded contradictory results. One of the studies showed no association between cancer and previous stressful events (Grisson et al., 1975). The other showed a significant correlation between cancer and loss of a loved person within the preceding five years (Horne and Picard, 1979). The latter finding is open to question, however, since age may have been a confounding variable. Two epidemiological studies – one in Britain (Jones et al., 1984) and one in Denmark (Ewertz, 1986) – found no association between breast cancer and previous loss of a spouse through death or divorce.

The suggested link between psychological stressors and the subsequent development of cancer is not demonstrated by the majority of controlled studies. In view of these results, and the fact that we cannot determine the exact date of onset of cancer, it would seem unprofitable to continue the search for a simple cause-and-effect relationship between stressful events and the onset of cancer.

It does not follow, however, that stress has no effect on the course of cancer. Investigations of that particular link do not suffer from the problem of being unable to date the onset of cancers. Local recurrence and the appearance of metastases can be dated with reasonable accuracy. Studies of the possible influence of stress on the progress of cancers have yielded some important results (see below). But such studies, which are as yet in their infancy, will need to use more sophisticated measures of stress than a simple enumeration of adverse life events. In particular, the effect of such events on the person as well as his or her specific coping responses should be measured.

Depression

Clinical observations from various sources have reported depression as a precursor of cancer. Systematic studies have produced conflicting results. In our own study of women with breast cancer (Greer and Morris, 1975), we found that almost identical proportions of cancer patients and control subjects with benign breast lumps had received treatment for depressive illness in the five years preceding the first appearance of the breast lump. Other researchers have studied cancer mortality in patients with depressive illness. Two studies reported higher-than-expected death rates from cancer in males with depressive illness, but two further studies found no such increase (Greer, 1983). These studies are, of course, subject to the same problem as that afflicting stress studies viz. that the date of onset of cancer is now known. It is possible that the frequently reported occurrence of depression preceding the clinical onset of cancer could be a symptom of early undetected malignant disease. In an attempt to overcome this difficulty, a large prospective investigation was undertaken by Shekelle *et al.* (1981) who gave psychological questionnaires to 2020 middle-aged males. Seventeen years later, the authors found a significant correlation between death from cancers and previous high depression scores. This study provides the most impressive evidence to date for a link between cancer and antecedent depression.

Personality traits

Since personality traits are supposedly life-long characteristics, the problem of dating the onset of cancer assumes less importance. The first controlled study was carried out by Kissen (1963) who compared male lung cancer patients with control subjects suffering from non-malignant, chronic lung diseases. He found a significant association between lung cancer and a reduced outlet for emotional discharge, i.e. an increased tendency to contain emotional conflict without any outward expression of this conflict. This personality trait was unrelated to cigarette consumption suggesting that 'both cigarette smoking and a characteristic personality type appear to be involved in the development of lung cancer' (Kissen, 1964).

In a later controlled study of women with breast cancer, Greer and Morris (1975) found a significant association between cancer and a behaviour pattern persisting during adult life of suppression of anger. An interesting subsidiary result emerged, viz. the association between suppression of anger and cancer reached statistical significance only in women under 50 years of age. Subsequently, several controlled studies of women with breast cancer have reported statistical correlations between cancer and emotional suppression (Scherg *et al.*, 1981; Wirsching *et al.*, 1982; Jansen and Muenz, 1984; Morris *et al.*, 1981). Three of these studies independently reported the same effect of age as in our original study. A controlled investigation of women with gynaecological cancers (mainly cervical, uterine, ovarian) revealed cancer patients to be significantly more controlled, more conforming and less aggressive than control

subjects with benign diseases (Mastrovito *et al.*, 1979).

Why are the reported correlations between breast cancer and emotional suppression only, or predominantly, applicable to younger patients? Fox, in an exhaustive critical review of the literature (Fox, 1978), put forward the following argument: cancers in children and young adults are, in all probability, mainly hereditary in origin, whereas cancers in elderly people are likely to arise through a combination of (a) increased exposure over many years to carcinogenic agents and (b) a greater susceptibility to cancer due to the presence of already transformed cells, impaired immune responses and other ageing processes. Consequently, he argued, any contribution of psychological factors to the development of cancer would be expected to be greatest in the middle years, perhaps 35 to 55. Fox's prediction is borne out by the reported results.

Although suppression of anger is the most consistently reported psychological correlate of cancer, suppression of anxiety has also been reported (Morris *et al.*, 1981; Magarey *et al.*, 1977; Kneier and Temoshok, 1984). This repressive coping style appears to be associated with physiological arousal as measured by electrodermal activity (skin conductance) (Kneier and Temoshok, 1984; Watson *et al.*, 1984). Hence, there is consistent evidence from a number of controlled studies that the development of certain cancers may be associated with a repressive coping style which has been called Type C personality.

It should be noted, however, that the evidence is based on studies that are either retrospective (i.e. obtained after the diagnosis is known) or quasi-prospective (i.e. obtained before the diagnosis is known but after clinical symptoms have appeared). Conclusive proof would require fully prospective studies in which healthy young adults are investigated psychologically and then followed up for 30 to 40 years to determine the incidence of cancer and its association with personality traits. It goes without saying that such studies are extremely difficult to carry out, not least because they demand longevity as well as extraordinary persistence on the part of the researcher. One such study is actually in progress (Thomas and McCabe, 1980); its final results are awaited with interest.

The evidence thus far points to a cancer-prone personality. This finding can be interpreted in two ways. First, there may be a genetic predisposition to the Type C personality as well as to certain cancers. The second interpretation is that these personality traits contribute to the development of cancer. Temoshok (1987) describes the Type C personality as characterized by suppression of negative feelings (especially anger), abrogation of one's needs in favour of others', being co-operative, unassertive, appeasing and accepting. She proposes that such traits result in a chronically blocked expression of needs and feelings which is likely to have adverse psychological and biological consequences. When faced with stressors, the Type C person suppresses feelings even more, leading to chronic but masked feelings of hopelessness and depression. The stage is set for the development of cancer. This speculative model proposed by Temoshok has the advantage of being empirically testable.

Conclusions

Further research is urgently required. Such research must be based on rigorous methodology. Future studies should involve large series of patients with a wide range of cancers at different stages of disease. Measures of suspected psychological prognostic factors should be reliable, valid and standardized on populations of cancer patients. The duration of follow-up should be as long as possible. Interactions between psychological and biological prognostic factors should be examined carefully. We remain profoundly ignorant, at present, about the specific physiological mechanisms which may mediate

psychological influences on tumour growth. Studies of physiological intermediary mechanisms are crucial for advances in knowledge in psycho-oncology.

References

Besedovski, H. and Sorkin, E. (1977) Hormonal control of immune processes. In James, V.H.T. (ed.) *Endocrinology Vol. 2 Proceedings V International Congress of Endocrinology*, 504–513, Excerpta Medica, Amsterdam–Oxford.

Burgess, C. (1978) Stress and cancer, *Cancer Surveys*, **6**, 403–416.

Cooper, C.L., Cooper, R. and Faragher, E.B. (1989) Incidence and perception of psychosocial stress: the relationship with breast cancer, *Psychol. Med.* **19**, 415–422.

Doll, R. and Peto, R. (1982) *The causes of cancer*, Oxford University Press, Oxford.

Ewertz, M. (1986) Bereavement and breast cancer, *Br. J. Cancer* **53**, 701–703.

Fox, B.H. (1978) Premorbid psychological factors as related to cancer incidence, *J. Behav. Med.* **1**, 45–133.

Greer, S. (1983) Cancer and the mind, *Br. J. Psychiat.*, **143**, 535–543.

Greer, S. and Brady, M. (1988) Natural Killer Cells: one possible link between cancer and the mind, *Stress Med.* **4**, 105–111.

Greer, S. and Morris, T. (1975) Psychological attributes of women who develop breast cancer: a controlled study, *J. Psychosom. Res.* **19**, 147–153.

Greer, S. and Morris, T. (1978) The study of psychological factors in breast cancer: problems of method, *Soc. Sci. Med.* **12**, 129–134.

Grisson, J.J., Weiner, B.J. and Weiner, E.A. (1975) Psychological correlates of cancer, *J. Cons. Clin. Psychol.* **43**, 113–117.

Guillemin, R., Vargo, I., Rossier, J., Minicks, S., Ling, N., Rivier, C., Vale, W. and Bloom, F. (1977) Beta-endorphins and adrenocorticotropin are secreted concomitantly by the pituitary gland, *Science* **197**, 1367–1369.

Herberman, R.B. (1981) Natural killer cells. In Sell, K.W. and Miller, W.V. (eds.) *The lymphocyte*, Liss, New York, 33–43.

Horne, R.L. and Picard, R.S. (1979) Psychosocial risk factors for lung cancers, *Psychosom. Med.* **41**, 503–514.

Irwin, J. and Asisman, H. (1984) Stress and pathology: immunological and central nervous system interactions. In Cooper, C.L. (ed.) *Psychosocial stress and cancer*, Wiley, Chichester, UK, 93–147

Jansen, M.A. and Muenz, L.R. (1984) A retrospective study of personality variables associated with fibrocystic disease and breast cancer, *J. Psychosom. Res.* **28**, 35–42.

Jones, D.R., Goldblatt, P.O. and Leon, D.A. (1984) Bereavement and cancer: some data on deaths of spouses from the longitudinal study of OPCS, *Br. Med. J.*, **289** 461–464.

Kissen, D.M. (1963) Personality characteristics in males conducive to lung cancer, *Br. J. Med. Psychol.* **36**, 27–36.

Kissen, D.M. (1964) Relationship between lung cancer, cigarette smoking, inhalation and personality, *Br. J. Med. Psychol.* **37**, 203–216.

Kneier, A.W. and Temoshok, L. (1984) Repressive coping reactions in patients with malignant emlanoma as compared to cardiovascular patients, *J. Psychosom. Res.* **28**, 145–155.

Le Shan, L. (1959) Psychological states as factors in the development of malignant disease: a critical review, *J. Natl. Cancer Inst.* **22**, 1–18.

Magarey, C.J., Todd, P.B. and Blizard, P.J. (1977) Psychosocial factors influencing delay and breast self-examination in women with symptoms of breast cancer, *Soc. Sci. Med.* **11**, 229–232.

Mastrovito, R.C., Deguire, K.S., Clarkin, J., Thaler, T., Lewis, J.L. and Cooper, E. (1979) Personality characteristics of women with gynaecological cancer, *Cancer Detection and Prevention* **2**, 281–287.

Mettler, C.C. and Mettler, H.W. (1947) *History of medicine*, Blakiston, Philadelphia.

Morris, T., Greer, S., Pettingale, K.W. and Watson, M. (1981) Patterns of expression of anger and their psychological correlates in women with breast cancer, *J. Psychosom. Res.* **25**, 111–117.

Muslin, H.L., Gyarfas, K. and Pieper, J. (1966) Separation experience and cancer of the breast, *N.Y. Acad. Sci.* 125, 802–806.

Pert, C.B., Ruff, M.R., Weber, R.J. and Herkenham, M. (1985) Neuropeptides and their receptors: a psychsomatic network, *J. Immunol.* **135**, 820–826.

Peters, L.J. and Mason, K.A. (1979) Influence of stress on experimental cancer. In Stoll, B. (ed.) *Mind and cancer prognosis*, Wiley, Chichester, UK, 103–124.

Pettingale, K.W. (1985) Towards a psychobiological model of cancer: biological considerations, *Soc. Sci. Med.* **20.**

Priestman, T.J., Priestman, S.G. and Bradshaw, C. (1985) Stress and breast cancer, *Br. J. Cancer* **51**, 493–498.

Razavi, D., Farvacques, C., Delcaux, N., Beffort, T., Paesmans, M., Leclercq, C., van Houtte, P. and Paridaens, R. (1990) Psychosocial correlates of oestrogen and progesterone receptors in breast cancer, *Lancet* **335**, 931–933.

Scherg, H., Cramer, I. and Blohmke, M. (1981) Psychosocial factors and breast cancer: a critical re-evaluation of established hypotheses, *Cancer Detection and Prevention*, **4**, 165–171.

Schonfield, J. (1975) Psychological and life experience differences between Israeli women with benign and cancerous breast lesions, *J. Psychosom. Res.* **19**, 229–234.

Shekelle, R.B., Raynor, W.J., Ostfeld, A.M., Garron, D.C., Bieliauskas, L.A., Liu, S.C., Maliza, C. and Oglesby, P. (1981) Psychosocial depression and 17-year risk of death from cancer, *Psychom. Med.* **43**, 117–125.

Stein, M., Keller, S. and Schleifer, S.J. (1985) Stress and immunomodulation: the role of depression and neuroendocrine function, *J. Immunol.*, **135**, 827–833.

Tecoma, E.S. and Huey, L.Y. (1985) Mini-review: psychic distress and the immune response, Life *Sciences* **36**, 1799–1812.

Temoshok, L. (1987) Personality, coping style, emotion and cancer: towards an integrative model, *Cancer Surv.* **6**, 545–567.

Thomas, C.B. and McCabe, O.L. (1980) Precursors of premature disease and death: habits of nervous tension, *John Hopkins Med. J.* **147**, 137–145.

Walshe, W.H. (1846) *The nature and treatment of cancer*, Taylor and Walton, London.

Watson, M., Pettingale, K.W. and Greer, S. (1984) Emotional control and autonomic arousal in breast cancer patients, *J. Psychosom. Res.* **28**, 467–474.

Wirsching, M., Stierlin, H., Hoffman, F., Weber, G. and Wirsching, B. (1982) Psychological identification of breast cancer patients before biopsy, *J. Psychosom. Res.* **26**, 1–10.

2 . 6

HORMONES AND CANCERS

Klim McPherson

Introduction

Hormones have effects which appear obscure and distant to their origin, and because they clearly affect growth as well as regulate other physiological processes they could, in principle, have unpredictable effects on cancers. This general concern is exacerbated by the increasing use of hormones in various medications. The publicity and apparent contradictions associating these hormone-based medications with cancer of various sites reflects both this concern and the real uncertainty surrounding the true nature of some of these associations.

This paper will discuss the evidence in the light of biological and epidemiological evidence. This will involve an understanding of the changing therapeutic use of different hormones, the development of biological research and the implications these have on the interpretation of the epidemiology.

What are hormones and what do they do?

Hormones are produced in one organ but generally have effects on distant target organs. They regulate a variety of physiological activities, such as reproduction and growth, as well as the maintenance of a stable internal environment.

It is thought that hormones have their effect on target organs via two main mechanisms. Firstly, by entering a target cell, the hormone can combine with an intracellular receptor protein, which together enters the cells' nucleus and affects the activity of specific genes. Because these genes carry the blueprint for protein synthesis, this can have far-reaching effects on the activities of cells.

Steroid hormones, including the sex hormones, are thought to act in this way.

The amino acid hormones, on the other hand, probably do not enter the target cell but combine with a receptor protein on the outer membrane of the cell. This complex then triggers an enzyme in the membrane causing the synthesis of a second compound which activates enzyme systems that bring about some action in the cell. Both mechanisms clearly depend on the binding of the hormone to a specific receptor molecule associated with the target cells. This is the mechanism whereby hormones are specific only to target cells which possess the particular receptor for that hormone.

As well as the action of **endogenous** hormones, i.e. those that are manufactured in the body for these normal processes, we also have to be concerned with the action of **exogenous** hormones, those that are taken for purposes such as contraception or hormone replacement therapy. We also need to be aware of the increasing environmental or dietary intake of hormones. Several cancers have at some time or another been suggested as having a cause which could in part possibly involve hormones (Armstrong, 1982), and these are shown in Table 1.

Table 1 Cancers in which hormones have been implicated

Salivary gland	Colon	Rectum
Liver	Gall-bladder	Pancreas
Breast	Cervix	Endometrium
Ovary	Prostate	Testis
Thyroid gland	Pituitary gland	

Mechanisms by which hormones may influence carcinogenesis

The process whereby cancer is caused is poorly understood in detail. Most analyses invoke some proposed or hypothetical biological mechanisms. Broadly, such processes involve modelling the division of cells in an organ up to the creation of a descendent cancerous cell. Such a cell will replicate and ultimately disseminate in an uncontrolled fashion. The process is called carcinogenesis.

In this process, a distinction is often made between initiation and promotion of cancer. **Initiation** involves the creation of cells which could in principle give rise to daughter cells which become cancer, while **promotion** is the process of conversion of initiated cells to cancer cells. The process of initiation is probably mutagenic and unlikely to be caused by hormones.

Moreover, the multi-stage model of cancer induction is more complex than simple initiation followed by promotion (Day, 1984). In this model the creation of a cancer cell happens as a result of several discrete stages or transitions, through which cell lines, destined to become cancer, have to pass. Thus to convert a cell line from one stage to another might require a particular kind of stimulus or exposure. Exposure to hormones might encourage, promote or affect the likelihood of transfer from some stages but not others.

Latent intervals between initiation, or early stage transformation, and the diagnosis of cancer may be decades in length and their actual duration may be characterized by considerable individual variation. An average latent interval of say 20 years may not be inconsistent with particular delays of just a few years. Weak evidence of a latent effect for a new exogenous hormonal exposure may be consistent with stronger subsequent delayed relationship.

The processes thus suggested are difficult to observe directly. Hence the demonstration, or indeed the refutation, of such a process is rarely straightforward. The combination of mathematical models and assiduous epidemiological study has enabled fairly strong conclusions to be made about the role of tobacco smoke in the carcinogenesis of lung cancer, but this is the most studied and understood carcinogenic process (Doll and Peto, 1981).

Studying hormones and cancer incidence

It is clear that providing evidence about hormones and cancer incidence that can reliably guide personal or public policy is extremely difficult. Individual measurements of hormone levels in the plasma are rarely undertaken. Even if they were, such information would not necessarily provide accurate information about levels in particular organs. Moreover, one might need to know the prevailing levels years before cancer is diagnosed. It is useless, for instance, to say that if a particular cancer seems to be hormonally dependent, all exogenous exposure to hormones should be avoided. Such exposure could as likely *protect* against the cancer as increase its incidence.

Evidence of a hormonal role in male cancers

Prostate cancer is the most common hormone-related male cancer. Little is actually known about its epidemiology. This cancer also does not occur in eunuchs, which suggests that androgens are important in its aetiology. Advanced prostate cancer is also effectively treated by the withdrawal of androgens, by castration. It also responds to the administration of oestrogen. One study has found that early puberty and greater sex drive are associated with an increase in incidence later in life, all of which supports an androgenic aetiology. Also men with cirrhosis, who have higher levels of circulating oestrogen, have lower prevalence of the disease.

In this disease it is clear that indirect observations of the associations give insight into its aetiology but do not provide very strong evidence for concrete understanding.

Evidence of a hormonal role in female cancers

Throughout Europe, the incidence of and mortality from cancer of the endometrium and the ovary are decreasing. In part this is because of the consistent finding in many epidemiological studies of a protective effect of oral contraceptive (OC) use. The incidence of cervical cancer and breast cancer is, on the other hand, increasing. Cervical cancer is increasing among the young, while breast cancer is increasing particularly among the elderly. Neither of these changes is likely to have very much to do with exogenous hormone use. The former is most likely to be a manifestation of changing sexual behaviour, while the latter is likely to be a consequence of general changes to do with diet, menstrual and other environmental influences, which may be mediated via hormones nonetheless.

Ovarian cancer

The incidence of cancer of the ovary increases with age progressively until about the time of the menopause, which strongly suggests a hormonal influence associated with ovarian function. However, it is more likely to be a function of repeated ovulation and hence indirectly related to hormones. This is supported by the observation that pregnancy, which suppresses ovulation, is protective.

It is also the case that three years' use of OCs decreases the risk of ovarian cancer by about a half, and that further use might decrease the risk by about 80%. This effect is seen soon after such OC use is completed and the protective effect is seen a long time after OCs have been discontinued (Doll and Peto, 1981). Thus, since OCs suppress ovulation quite successfully, such an effect is consistent with the theory that it is the trauma to the ovary associated with ovulation that is related to the risk of cancer. The trauma is followed by rapid cell growth which, in turn, gives rise to a higher risk. This would appear to be an indirect effect of hormones.

Endometrial cancer

Endometrial cancer is increased by unopposed (oestrogen only) hormonal replacement therapy (HRT). During menstruation unopposed endogenous oestrogen is responsible for endometrial proliferation during the first half of the cycle. Subsequent exposure during the second half to progesterone inhibits this proliferation.

Exposure to combined oral contraceptives for 21 days in a cycle should be expected to reduce the risk of endometrial cancer because fewer cycles during life will have been exposed to unopposed oestrogen. Likewise the addition of progesterone to HRT (opposed therapy) should be associated with no increase in risk. The epidemiology tells us that there is around half the risk among women who have used OCs for three or more years. One reliable study has reported a 70% reduction in risk 15 years after OCs were discontinued. It is possible, however, that sequential preparations increase the risk of endometrial cancer. There is no doubt that opposed HRT has little or no effect on endometrial cancer risk, in contrast to the effect of unopposed HRT.

Cervical cancer

The evidence for an effect of endogenous oestrogens on cervical cancer is weak. This cancer can however be induced in mice by exposure to oestrogens and progestogens. Examination of the age–incidence curve of this disease is difficult to interpret because of cohort changes in incidence associated with changing sexual habits and the relationship between sexual maturity and sexual activity. Cervical cancer is most strongly related to the number of male sexual partners and also to the number of partners each partner has had. It is therefore probably sexually transmitted, most likely by a virus.

The epidemiology of cervical cancer is a difficult disease to study because of several factors. Since sexual habits are often related to the use of endogenous hormones and may be dependent upon the amount and extent of OC exposure, it can be difficult to disentangle physiology from contraceptive choices on the cellular effects seen on the cervix. Several studies indicate that barrier methods of contraception, such as the diaphragm and the condom, reduce the risk of cervical cancer or pre-cancer and hence any control group against whom hormone users may be compared have to be studied carefully.

Cervical smears are in general more likely to be taken from young women if they are OC users, simply because OC users will be in contact with primary care services more often. Hence pre-invasive lesions, which have been allowed to progress, will appear to be more common among users of contraceptive methods that do not require frequent medical visits. It is also possible that cigarette-smoking is related to an increased risk of cervical cancer, but smoking may be related to contraceptive choice and hence any causative pathway is again confused.

In spite of all these problems, most studies do show an increase in risk associated with long-term OC use after all the proper adjustments have been made. Approximately a doubling of risk compared to other non-barrier methods after around eight years of use is a typical finding. Such an effect, because it is so small, will always be confused with the possibility that it is merely the manifestation of the kind of biases already discussed.

Breast cancer

The importance of ovarian hormones, and in particular oestrogens, in the genesis of breast cancer has long been established. Their influence on the risk of breast cancer was first suggested in 1836. It was observed that the stage of the menstrual cycle influenced the rate of breast-tumour cell proliferation. However, it was not until the late 19th-century experiments of Beatson that any direct supporting evidence was provided (Beatson, 1886); women with advanced breast cancer were observed to go into remission after oophorectomy. Animal experiments have also tended to point to ovarian dependence of breast tumours, with oestrogens in particular having been observed to induce breast cancer in a variety of species.

Breast cancer is thus unequivocally hormonally related. This has led to enormous concern surrounding the role of exogenous hormones on the risk of this common disease, which has a lifetime risk of around 6%.

Oestrogens are administered today either for contraception or for treatment of menopausal symptoms. The combined oral contraceptive pill consists of one of the two synthetic oestradiol-17B derivatives ethinyl oestradiol or its 3-methyl ether mestranol, and one of a number of progestogens. Menopausal hormone replacement therapy (HRT) primarily employs conjugated equine oestrogen either with or without accompanying progestogen.

Hormone replacement therapy

It is widely accepted that long-term, high-dose, menopausal oestrogen administration is associated with a modest increase in breast-cancer risk. The first epidemiological study to point to such an association was a cohort study published in the mid-1970s by Hoover *et al.* (1976). A dose–response relationship was observed with the relative risk for 15 years' use reaching 2.0. Additionally, after 10 years of follow-up, HRT was observed to remove the protective influence of oophorectomy, as was also observed later by others. A number of case-control and cohort studies followed, most of which detected a modest increase in risk for HRT use, although not all observed a dose–response relationship, and some raised relative risks were confined to subgroups only.

This lack of consistency could be attributable to heterogeneity of study design. It has recently been estimated that the relative risk of 20 years' HRT use might be around 1.75 (Hulka, 1990). Other recent cohort studies confirm this estimate, although this risk could be as great as double for 15 years of use. Current studies, moreover, are unable to reliably distinguish any different effect of the addition of progestogens in opposed therapy. The epidemiology, however, seems to suggest that the effect of HRT use per year on breast-cancer risk is less than an equivalent natural delay in menopause would have been. This is presumably because the dose of hormone to which the breast is exposed is less than the exposure attributable to normal ovarian function. Moreover, this effect is seen soon after accumulating the HRT exposure, suggesting an effect on a late stage of carcinogenesis.

Oral contraceptives

Studying large groups of contraceptive users in cohort studies, which were mostly begun in the sixties, soon after OCs became available, have shown little cause for concern. Long-term OC use has hardly been shown to be associated with any change in breast-cancer risk. Only one cohort study has reported an elevated risk for women who have ever used OCs – for breast cancer, at a young age. A useful review of the evidence by Prentice and Thomas shows a relative risk of (essentially) unity for long-term OC use and breast-cancer risk (Prentice and Thomas, 1987).

Several recent case-control studies, in which breast-cancer cases are compared with controls without the disease, appear to show an association between OC use at a young age and breast cancer. These studies are not unanimous; some others seem to show no association. These discrepancies may be, in part, attributable to survey biases inherent in observational case-control study methodology.

The epidemiology of breast cancer shows three features to be particularly relevant in the interpretation of the epidemiology. Firstly, a young age at menarche is a risk factor for the disease. Because breast cancer is very uncommon until the mid-forties, early menarche must therefore be associated with an elapsed interval of at least 20 years. Secondly, in the follow-up study of survivors of the atomic bombs in Hiroshima and Nagasaki, teenage girls were observed to have a dose-related increased risk of breast cancer. However, none was diagnosed in the first 10 years of follow-up and this effect was not finally demonstrated until 20 or more years after exposure. Radiation is a known carcinogen, however, and hence probably affects initiation.

Thirdly, in studies of the effect of diethylstilbestrol (DES), a non-steroidal hormone introduced in the 1940s and 50s to prevent miscarriage, an association has been shown between its use and breast-cancer incidence. One such study of 3,000 exposed women and 3,000 similar women who were not exposed to the drug showed a relative risk of around 2 associated with exposure (Greenbury et al., 1984). This was after some 40 years of follow-up, but after 20 years there was no divergence at all in the cumulative risk curves. This gives rise to the particular concern that DES might affect some early part of the carcinogenic process in the breast, which is associated with a long latent period.

Since age at first full-term pregnancy is a strong risk factor for the disease, an early first pregnancy being protective, it is possible that

OC use before first pregnancy could have an effect not seen with OC use afterwards.

On the basis of evidence from cancer registration there is clearly no strong immediate effect of OCs, because if there were, then it would have appeared in cancer registrations by now. However, it is not possible to derive much reassurance from the observed lack of change, if there is a long latent effect. The pill is now so popular that the kind of effect we have been discussing could have serious consequences on breast-cancer risk later this century and unfortunately current epidemiology cannot yet convincingly refute such ideas.

Overall effects of hormonal administration

A balanced view must take account of the protective effect of the pill on endometrial and ovarian cancer. A halving of the risk of these cancers among every user of OCs would reduce the lifetime incidence by about 11 new cases per 1,000. Such a reduction would be balanced by an ultimate relative risk of breast cancer of around only 1.3 associated with four or so years of early use, because breast cancer is so much more common. If this relative risk is higher than that then the net effect of OCs will be to increase overall cancer incidence.

Calculations of the overall benefits and risks of OCs including mortality from all diseases known to be associated with their administration suggests that OC users will have fewer deaths between the ages of 16 and 50. However, if breast cancer does have the kind of relationship with OCs postulated here into middle age then this protection will be swamped (Vessey, 1990).

Similarly, with respect to the administration of HRT, the unambiguous benefit on osteomalacia and the possible benefit of therapy on coronary heart disease lead to the possibility of an overall benefit. However, these beneficial effects of opposed (in contrast to unopposed) therapy on the risk of cardiovascular disease and cerebrovascular disease are not yet conclusively established. The breast-cancer risk is clearly only important after very long-term use of HRT. As with much of this evidence, its resolution awaits definitive work once the period between long-term exposure and possible disease is sufficiently studied among a large number of women.

References

Armstrong, B. (1982) Endocrine factors in human carcinogenesis. In Bartch, H. and Armstrong, B. (eds.) *Host factors in human carcinogenesis*, IARC, Lyon, 93–221.

Beatson, G.T. (1886) On the treatment of inoperable cases of carcinoma of the mamma, *Lancet* ii:104–107.

Day. N.E. (1984) *Epidemiological data and multi-stage carcinogenesis*, IARC Sci. Publ. 56, IARC, Lyon.

Doll, R. and Peto, R. (1981) *The causes of cancer*, Oxford University Press, Oxford.

Greenberg, E.R., Barnes, A.B., Ressequie, L. *et al.* (1984) Breast cancer in mother given diethylstibestrol in pregnancy, *New Engl. J. Med* **311** 1393–1397.

Hoover, R., Gray, L.A., Cole, P. and McMahon, B. (1976) Menopausal oestrogens and breast cancer, *N. Engl. J. Med.* **295** 401–405.

Hulka, B. (1990) Hormone replacement therapy and the risk of breast cancer, *CA* **40**, No. 5, 289–296.

Prentice, R.L. and Thomas, D.B. (1987) On the epidemiology of oral contraceptives and disease, *Adv. Cancer Research* **49**, 285–401.

Vessey, M.P. (1990) An overview of the benefits and risks of combined oral contraceptives, In *Oral Contraceptives and Breast Cancer*, Mann, R.D. (ed.) Parthenon Publishing Group, Lancashire, United Kingdom.

TOBACCO AND CANCERS

E. Heseltine, E. Riboli, L. Shuker and J. Wilbourn

Tobacco production and use

Smoking tobacco

Tobacco was first smoked by the native populations of North America; after tobacco was brought to Europe in the middle of the sixteenth century, smoking spread throughout the world, particularly after 1918 when the cigarette industry began expanding.

By the early 1980s, over 4 million hectares of tobacco were under cultivation world-wide, with a total production in 1982 of over 6.5 million tonnes. In Europe, 510,046 hectares of tobacco were cultivated in 1982, yielding 760,086 tonnes. International trade in raw tobacco was about 1.5 million tonnes annually.

In developed countries tobacco is most widely smoked in the form of cigarettes, although in the early lives of a lot of the population at risk today tobacco was taken in the form of cigars and pipe tobacco. Cigarettes are made from fine-cut tobaccos blended with varying proportions of different grades of Virginia and other tobaccos. In northern Europe cigarettes made entirely of Virginia tobacco are preferred, whereas in France and southern Europe cigarettes filled with dark, air-cured tobaccos are more popular.

Cigarette design has changed significantly over the past few decades, due to demands for lower yields of certain smoke components (especially total particulate matter and nicotine), largely in response to a growing concern about the adverse health effects associated with tobacco smoking. The major changes in cigarette design include more specific blend selection, variations in length and circumference, addition of filters, the use of reconstituted tobacco sheet and expanded tobacco, and the development of ventilation techniques.

The standard laboratory methods for determining the yields of particulate matter ('tar' and nicotine) cannot faithfully represent human smoking practices and thus have limited applicability in relation to specific human dosage. However, major reductions in the measured levels of tar have been achieved by altering the design of filter tips. The popularity of filter-tipped cigarettes increased markedly from the early 1950s, after the publication of studies demonstrating a causal relationship between smoking and lung cancer. In 1982 filter cigarettes accounted for 90% or more of the cigarette market in many countries. In Europe exceptions to this trend are seen in the USSR, where only 30% of cigarettes are sold filter-tipped, Poland with 45%, France with 47% and the Netherlands with 67%. Filtered types have significantly less dry particulate matter than non-filter cigarettes, although carbon monoxide delivery may be higher.

Before filter tips began to be widely used, typical tar deliveries were generally more than 30 mg per cigarette. Even in countries where no systematic effort has been made to reduce tar deliveries, values in the range 20–30 mg are now typical; whereas in countries where substantial reductions have been deliberately engendered, the average tar delivery is now likely to be under 15 mg. However, tar and nicotine yields of commercial cigarettes vary widely around the world. In 1983 cigarettes delivering more than 30 mg of tar were still sold in many countries, including Austria, China, France, Hong Kong, India, Indonesia, Italy, Kenya, the Philippines, Scotland, South Africa and the USSR.

Estimates of world tobacco consumption show it rising in most countries between 1920 and the 1960s. The rise is occasionally interrupted by major events such as war, financial depression or reports by health bodies, such as the US Surgeon General and the Royal College of Physicians in the UK. In some countries, such as Finland, the UK and the USA, cigarette consumption per person has been declining in recent years. Smokers generally represent between one third and one half of the adult male population of a country – Japan, with a higher proportion – is one of the few exceptions in the developed world. In most countries, about one third of the adult women smoke. Smoking rates among adolescents, although of considerable importance to public health as an indication of future trends, are extremely difficult to measure accurately. It is usual for smoking habits to become established during adolescence, and the smoking rates of people in their late teens may approximate or be greater than those of adults.

Smokeless tobacco

Faced with the threat of potentially declining cigarettes sales, resulting from wider knowledge of the health consequences of smoking and from public concern about risks due to passive smoking, the tobacco industry has expressed a renewed interest in so-called 'smokeless' tobacco products.

In Europe and the US, the smokeless tobacco products are mainly chewing tobacco and snuff. The categorization of products into one of these two classes is not clear, and there appears to be considerable overlap, depending on national legislation. For instance in the US some types of fine-cut smokeless tobacco, classified as chewing tobacco before 1981, are now categorized as moist/fine-cut snuff.

Chewing tobaccos can either be chewed or portions can be placed between the inside of the lip and the gums for varying periods. Like chewing tobacco, snuff can be used orally by placing it between the inside of the lip and the gums. Most snuff used today has a relatively high moisture content and is finely cut rather than pulverized. Dry, pulverised forms of

snuff are predominantly used orally, although nasal sniffing is still practised.

A 1978 estimate indicated 700,000 to 800,000 snuff users in Sweden (about 17% of the population); almost all of whom were men. Among Swedish school children aged 13–16 years, 11–15% of boys took snuff regularly, Use of oral snuff is also widespread in Denmark. Estimates of the number of current users of smokeless tobacco worldwide range from 7–22 million people.

Recently, oral tobacco products such as *Skoal Bandits* have appeared on the market. These fine-cut, moist tobacco mixtures are placed in containers similar to tea-bags and are sold in varying strengths of nicotine with a choice of flavourings. The packaging and logos of these products and their aggressive advertising campaigns are directed toward young male users, although this intention is denied by the industry. Their use is associated with sports figures, thereby implying that they pose no threat to health and may be a good substitute for cigarette smoking in areas where smoking is prohibited.

Constituents of tobacco smoke

The burning of tobacco produces yields mainstream smoke and sidestream smoke. Mainstream smoke, which is generated in the burning cone and hot zones when the cigarette is drawn, travels through the tobacco column and exits from the mouthpiece. Sidestream smoke forms between drawing and is emitted into the air freely from the smouldering tobacco product.

Tobacco smoke contains more than 3900 chemical constituents; concentrations range from nanograms to milligrams per cigarette. Many of these components have been evaluated for carcinogenicity by IARC working groups (see Table 1).

Table 1 Chemicals in tobacco smoke associated with cancers

Chemicals identified in tobacco smoke that are causally associated with cancer in humans

4-Aminobiphenyl	Chromium (hexavalent compounds)
Arsenic	Nickel
Benzene	Vinyl chloride

Chemicals identified in tobacco smoke that are probably carcinogenic to humans

Benzo[a]pyrene	Formaldehyde
Cadmium	N-Nitrosodiethylamine
Dibenz[a,h]anthracene	N-Nitrosodimethylamine

Chemicals identified in tobacco smoke for which there are inadequate or no data on carcinogenicity in humans, but for which sufficient evidence exists of carcinogenicity in experimental animals

Acetaldehyde	Indeno [1,2,3-cd]pyrene
Benzo[b]fluoranthene	Lead (inorganic)
Benzo[j]fluoranthene	5-Methylchrysene
Benzo[k]fluoranthene	2-Nitropropane
para-cresol	N-Nitrosodi-n-butylamine
DDT	N-Nitrosodiethanolamine
Dibenz[a,h]acridine	N-Nitrosodi-n-propylamine
Dibenz [a,j]acridine	4-(N-Nitrosomethylamino)-1-(3-pyridyl)-1-butanone
7-H-Dibenzo[c,g]carbazole	N-Nitrosomethylethyamine
Dibenzo[a,e]pyrene	N'-Nitrosonornicotine
Dibenzo[a,h]pyrene	N-Nitrosopiperidine
Dibenzo[a,f]pyrene	N-Nitrosopyrrolidine
Dibenzo[a,i]pyrene	ortho-Toluidine
Hydrazine	Urethane

Tobacco smoke's major toxic effects, other than cancers, are caused by the presence of carbon monoxide, nitrogen oxides, ammonia, hydrogen cyanide and acrolein in tobacco smoke .

The majority of the mutagenic and carcinogenic agents reside in the particulate phase. Tar is not a separate agent but is defined as that portion of cigarette smoke retained on a special filter, minus water and nicotine. Tar is a complex mixture of chemicals, many of which can cause cancers in laboratory animals.

Nonsmokers are exposed to effluents comprising both sidestream and mainstream smoke expelled by active smokers.

Mainstream smoke is inhaled almost undiluted whereas sidestream smoke is considerably diluted in the air. However sidestream smoke has been shown to contain greater amounts of identified carcinogens than mainstream smoke.

Constituents of smokeless tobacco

At least 2500 chemical constituents have been identified in unburnt tobacco. This number includes the tobacco constituents themselves, as well as chemicals applied to tobacco during cultivation, harvesting and processing. The classes of compounds identified in tobacco include all the major types of organic chemical.

The tobacco-specific N-nitrosamines – N'-nitrosonornicotine (NNN), NNK, N'-nitrosoanatabine (NAT) and N-nitrosoanabasine (NAB) – are the only identified carcinogens that occur in mg/kg concentrations. Microgram per kilogram levels of some carcinogenic polynuclear aromatic hydrocarbons and metal compounds and of the α-emitting polonium-210 have also been detected.

Processed tobacco contained 27 volatile amines, 11 aromatic amines and more than 50 N-heterocyclic compounds, such as pyrroles, pyrrolidines, imidazoles, pyridines and pyrazines. Of special relevance to tobacco carcinogenesis are secondary amines, which can give rise to N-nitrosamines during curing, fermentation and ageing. Compounds containing nitrogen, including nitrates, amines, amides and proteins, comprise up to 24% of cured and fermented tobaccos, from which many smokeless tobacco products are made. Some of these compounds are known precursors of N-nitrosamines. A large number of studies have shown that during the ageing, curing, fermentation and processing of tobacco, nicotine and other alkaloids give rise to carcinogenic, tobacco-specific N-nitrosamines. The concentration of these

compounds in tobacco exceeds by at least 100 times the concentrations found so far in other products, such as cured meat, whisky and beer. It has been calculated that in the US cigarette smoking gives rise to at least a 20-fold daily exposure to N-nitroso compounds than any other product.

However, since the relative concentration of NNN, NNK and NAT in chewing tobacco is much greater than in cigarette smoke, and since the average chewer consumes 10 g of tobacco compared with just over 1 g tar inhaled by the smoker, tobacco chewing appears to be the greatest exogenous source of exposure to N-nitrosamines.

Tobacco smoking and cancers

In 1950 five papers appeared in the UK and the US describing studies in which the smoking habits of large numbers of patients with cancer of the lung or, in some studies, with cancers of the mouth, pharynx or larynx, were compared with the smoking habits of control patients. One of these studies concluded that 'smoking is a factor, and an important factor, in the production of carcinoma of the lung' (Doll and Hill, 1950).

The conclusions drawn from these studies were checked by recording the smoking habits of large numbers of men and women who smoked different amounts and following them over several years to find whether the recorded habits helped in predicting the risk of disease developing. This method, moreover, allowed for study not only of the relationship between smoking and lung cancer, but also of that between smoking and other cancers and all other diseases where a substantial number of cases occurred within the period of observation.

Many such studies have now been carried out, eight of which cover enough individuals for a long enough period for useful information to be obtained about a wide range of diseases. On the basis of these and of other smaller studies, conclusions can be drawn about the strength of the association between smoking and cancers at different sites.

Lung cancer

Lung cancer is believed to be the most common fatal neoplastic disease in the world today, and the overall pattern is one of rapid increase. Three factors are contributing to this continuing increase. First, increased access to diagnosis and progressive improvements in the accuracy of certification of cause of death mean that an increasing proportion of fatal lung cancers are recognized as such. Second, the number of adults old enough to be at risk of developing the disease is increasing rapidly. Finally, and most importantly, large increases in the numbers of people smoking cigarettes are producing large increases in age-specific lung cancer rates. Most of this increase is the result of the growth in cigarette smoking by young adults in the second half of this century.

Most cases of lung cancer result from tobacco smoking. In populations where prolonged widespread cigarette smoking began several decades ago, it generally accounts for more than 80% of cases (and for more than 90% in males). In populations where the effect of smoking has yet to peak – among young adults and most female populations – the proportion may currently be lower.

The high proportion of lung cancer cases due to smoking does not preclude the possibility that other carcinogenic factors may contribute to the total . For example, in populations which experienced heavy industrial development during this century, joint exposures to tobacco smoke and occupational carcinogens may account for up to 10–30% of all cases of lung cancer.

The observed relationship between tobacco smoking and the incidence of lung cancer appears to depend on four factors.

1 **The daily dose of tobacco**. Findings consistently show that, among otherwise similar cigarette smokers, a direct, often linear, relationship exists between the daily dose of tobacco and the excess risk of lung cancer in both men and women.

2 **The duration of regular smoking**. Because damage to the lung accumulates with continual smoking, the incidence of lung cancer depends strongly on the duration of smoking. People who start to smoke in adolescence and who continue to smoke as adults are at the greatest risk of developing lung cancer in adult life. The relationship between the age at which regular cigarette smoking started and lung cancer death rates at the age of 55–64 years for men in the US is shown in Figure 1. Studies in many countries show a delay of several decades between the widespread adoption of cigarette smoking by young adults and the emergence of its full effects on national lung cancer rates.

People who have been smoking for many years (who have not already developed lung cancer or some other disease) can reduce the risk of tobacco-induced lung cancer by ceasing to smoke. When smoking ceases, the annual excess risk of developing lung cancer appears to remain roughly constant for many years thereafter. Thus, after smoking for 15 years, the annual excess incidence of lung cancer is approximately 0.005%, or 5 per 100 000; after 30 years it is about 0.1%, or 1 per 1000; and after 45 years it is about 0.5%, or 5 per 1000. If a smoker stops after smoking for 30 years, 15 years later the annual excess risk may still be about 0.1%, instead of the 0.5% it would have been if smoking had continued. Stopping smoking avoids about 80% of the excess risk associated with continued smoking.

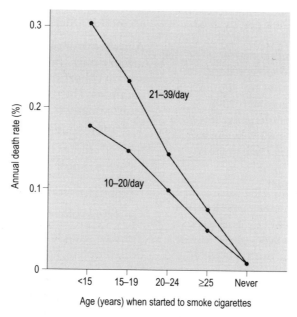

Figure 1   Relationship between age of starting regular cigarette smoking in early adult life and lung cancer death rates at age 55-64 (mean 60) for men in the United States; data presented separately for heavy and for moderate smokers.

Source: Doll and Peto (1981)

3 **The form in which tobacco is smoked (cigarettes, cigars, pipes).** Findings show that, among otherwise similar smokers, those who use only cigarettes have much higher lung cancer risks than those who used only pipes and/or cigars, although pipe and cigar smoking cause some appreciable risk. The estimated risk to pipe and cigar smokers appears to be lie between the risks to cigarette smokers and nonsmokers.

4 **The type of cigarette smoked.** Soon after the lung cancer risks from smoking (especially cigarette smoking) were established in the 1950s, cigarettes were substantially modified in some countries. At present no direct comparison of the health effects of lifelong use of modified and unmodified cigarettes is possible. However, although adequate cohort studies are not yet available to assess whether changes in the composition of cigarettes (e.g. use of filters, reduction in tar level)

have modified the risk of lung cancer from *prolonged* use of such cigarettes, some conclusions about current use can be drawn from available data.

In one large cohort study, cigarettes delivering less than 17.6mg of tar were associated with a lower risk for lung cancer than were those delivering more than 25.7mg of tar. In other epidemiological studies, there was a fairly consistent tendency for lung cancer risks to be lower among users of filter cigarettes than of non-filter cigarettes. The reduction seen in the largest and most recent study was about 40-50%, which was statistically highly significant. In that study, tar yields were also recorded and found to be positively associated with lung cancer risk.

In a few countries where changes in cigarette design and composition began in the late 1950s or early 1960s, cigarette smoking by men had been established so many years previously that the lung cancer rates in early middle-aged men had largely or wholly completed their rise by 1960. They might have been expected to remain approximately constant thereafter if the risk per cigarette had remained constant, however, a few years after the significant changes in cigarette manufacturing (associated with reductions in tar levels), a decrease in lung cancer rates began to appear in these particular age groups.

Cancers of the urinary tract

Major cohort studies and many case-control studies in various parts of the world have consistently associated cancers of the lower urinary tract (renal pelvis, ureter, bladder and urethra), and specifically cancers of the bladder and renal pelvis with cigarette smoking. These studies generally show a dose-response relationship for men, with risks for those smoking the largest number of cigarettes per day being about five times greater than those for nonsmokers. Such conclusions can not be drawn with regard to women, due to smaller case numbers and less prolonged smoking.

Duration of cigarette smoking was shown to be directly related to the risk for bladder cancer in men. When cancers of the renal pelvis and of the ureter were considered separately, a dose-response relationship with daily or cumulative consumption of tobacco was found, with risks generally higher than those for cancer of the bladder. Pipe smoking and cigar smoking probably also increase the risk for bladder cancer, but at lower levels than cigarette smoking.

The proportion of bladder cancers in the general population that can be attributed to cigarette smoking has been calculated in several studies. These show that in most countries with a history of prolonged cigarette use, 50% of male cases and 25% of female cases of bladder cancer are attributable to smoking. No other independently important

factor, such as occupation, has been shown to account for this association.

A lowering of risk for cancers of the lower urinary tract after stopping smoking has been seen in cohort studies carried out in many countries. The risk of ex-smokers thus approximates that of nonsmokers more than 15 years after giving up smoking.

Several studies have also shown an association between cancer of the kidney and cigarette smoking.

Cancers at other sites

Tobacco smoking is an important cause of oral, oropharyngeal, hypopharyngeal, laryngeal and oesophageal cancers, and the risk increases with increasing tobacco use. The risk grows substantially when cigarette smoking is combined with heavy consumption of alcohol. Pipe smoking and cigar smoking appear to increase the risk for these cancers to approximately the same extent as cigarette smoking does. Tobacco smokers also appear to run increased risks of cancer of the lip.

Epidemiological studies of various types consistently point to tobacco smoking as an important cause of pancreatic cancer. No other factor that could explain this relationship has been identified.

The higher risks seen among tobacco smokers for cancers of the stomach, liver and cervix cannot be attributed with certainty to smoking, since in none of the studies has it been possible to rule out other factors.

For cancer of the endometrium, many studies have shown slightly lower risks for women who smoke cigarettes. This weak negative association may be related to the detrimental effect of smoking in reducing the age at which menopause occurs, and does not provide any material advantage to smokers. With regard to breast cancer, a number of studies have shown no consistent effect of smoking on risk.

Interactions with other factors in causing cancers

Studies of tobacco smokers who are exposed to certain other agents show that the tobacco-smoking segment of the population runs substantially greater risks of cancers than the risks experienced by the general population. Some of the most prominent groups are alcohol drinkers, workers exposed to asbestos and people exposed to ionizing radiation in uranium mines. Exposure to these agents increases the risk of cancers.as it has been shown that they have an almost multiplicative interaction with smoking.

The enhanced risk from drinking alcohol is dose-dependent, and the risk, relative to that for nonsmoking nondrinkers, increases almost multiplicatively with an increasing level of alcohol consumption. This relationship is observed for cancers of the oral cavity, oropharynx, hypopharynx and oesophagus.

The pattern that emerges from studies of asbestos workers is of an interaction between occupational exposure to asbestos varieties and tobacco smoking. In insulators, the joint effect is multiplicative. A multiplicative effect with cigarette smoking was also seen for uranium miners exposed to radioactive alpha emissions in mines in the US.

Tobacco habits other than smoking

The oral and nasal use of tobacco, either finely powdered as snuff or in leaf form for chewing, is as old as its use for smoking in pipes, cigars and cigarettes. In the first half of the twentieth century, the use of chewing tobacco and snuff in the western hemisphere was overtaken by a huge increase in the use of smoking tobacco. In some parts of the world, however, including the Indian subcontinent, south-east

Asia and much of the Middle East, smokeless tobacco is still widely used. Additionally, chewing tobacco and snuff have enjoyed a renaissance in western countries during recent years.

Epidemiological studies carried out in Europe and North America clearly show that the use of smokeless tobacco products is associated with an increased risk for contracting cancer of the mouth. Since the design of these studies differs widely, it would be cumbersome to try to tabulate them, however certain clear associations emerge. In most of the studies no distinction was made between chewing tobacco and snuff as the difference between the two is blurred, relating mainly to the fineness of the product. Moreover, categorization of the two types has changed recently, at least in the US, thus chewing tobacco is described as such in only a few studies. Oral use of snuff, on the other hand, has been related consistently with cancers of the oral cavity and pharynx. In addition, cancers frequently developed at the site at which snuff was habitually applied.

Studies that have not distinguished snuff from chewing tobacco are informative for three reasons, when considered with other studies. First, reports of oral cancer cases confirm the high relative frequency of the use of smokeless tobacco products among patients; other studies report that use of smokeless tobacco is moderately to strongly associated with oral cancer. Second, a dose-response relationship was found in one large study in which the risks for oral cancer in men ranged from four-fold for moderate use of smokeless tobacco to more than six-fold with heavy use. Lastly two large studies provide evidence of a positive association with cancers. One study showed a two-fold to three-fold increase in risk of death from oral, pharyngeal and oesophageal cancer; the second study indicated a similar increase from oesophageal cancer.

References

Doll, R. (1986) Tobacco: an overview of health effects. In Zaridze, D. and Peto, R. (eds.) *Tobacco. A major international health hazard*, IARC scientific publications, No. 74, International Agency for Research on Cancer, Lyon, 11-22.

Doll, R. and Peto, R.(1981) *The causes of cancer*, Oxford University Press

Hoffmann, D., Wynder, E.L. (1986) Chemical constituents and bioactivity of tobacco smoke. In Zaridze, D. and Peto, R. (eds.) *Tobacco. A major international health hazard*, IARC scientific publications, no. 74, International Agency for Research on Cancer, Lyon, 145-165.

IARC (1985) IARC monographs on the evaluation of the carcinogenic risk of chemicals to humans, vol. 37, *Tobacco habits other than smoking; betel-quid and areca-nut chewing; and some related nitrosamines*, International Agency for Research on Cancer, Lyon.

IARC (1986) IARC monographs on the evaluation of the carcinogenic risk of chemicals to humans, vol. 38, *Tobacco smoking*, International Agency for Research on Cancer, Lyon.

IARC (1987) IARC monographs on the evaluation of the carcinogenic risk of chemicals to humans, suppl. 7, *Overall evaluations of carcinogenicity:* an updating of IARC monographs volumes 1 to 42, International Agency for Research on Cancer, Lyon.

Murphy, J.F. (1984) The effects of material smoking on the unborn child. In Studd, J. (ed.) *Progress in obstetrics and gynaecology,* Churchill Livingstone, Edinburgh, 36-51.

O'Neill, I.K. *et al,* (1987) (eds.) Environmental carcinogens. Methods of analysis and exposure measurement, vol. 9. In: *Passive smoking,*.IARC scientific publications, no. 81, International Agency for Research on Cancer, Lyon.

Paffenbarger, R. S. Jr. *et al.*(1986) Cigarette smoking and cardiovascular diseases. In Zaridze, D. and Peto, R. (eds.) *Tobacco. A major international health hazard*, IARC scientific publications, no. 74, International Agency for Research on Cancer Lyon, 45-60.

Peach, H. (1986) Smoking and respiratory disease excluding lung cancer. In Zaridze, D. and Peto, R. (eds.) *Tobacco. A major international health hazard*, IARC scientific publications, no. 74, International Agency for Research on Cancer Lyon, 61-72.

Saracci, R., Riboli, E. (1992) Passive smoking and lung cancer: current evidence and ongoing studies at the International Agency for Research on Cancer. *Mutation research* [in press].

Sasco, A. J. (1987).*Rapport préliminaire sur la législation en vigueur pour l'étiquetage des produits du tabac et la limite en goudrons des cigarettes dans les pays de la Communauté Economique Européene*, International Agency for Research on Cancer, Lyon.

Stellman, S. D. (1986) Influence of cigarette yield on risk of coronary heart disease and chronic obstructive lung disease. In: Zaridze, D. and Peto, R. (eds.) *Tobacco. A major international health hazard*, IARC scientific publications, no. 74, International Agency for Research on Cancer, Lyon, 237-249.

Wald, N. *et al.* (1992) *UK smoking statistics*, Oxford University Press, Oxford [in press].

PASSIVE SMOKING

Martin J. Jarvis

Introduction

Concern about passive smoking as a health issue is surprisingly recent. The term itself appears to date from 1970 and it was not until 1982 that interest was widely aroused, with the publication of reports from Japan and Greece that non-smoking women married to smokers are at increased risk for lung cancer (Hirayama, 1981; Trichopoulos *et al.*, 1981). Since then, there has been a veritable explosion of activity both on the research front and by campaigners seeking to protect non-smokers from having to breathe other people's smoke. The tobacco industry, for its part, has made it clear that it sees passive smoking as a key issue determining the future social acceptability of the smoking habit, and has vigorously combated the emerging evidence of health effects and has sought instead to portray the matter as one simply of good manners (Tobacco Advisory Council, 1989a; Tobacco Advisory Council, 1989b).

This paper will begin by summarizing the evidence that passive smoking is harmful to non-smokers' health. In so doing, it will attempt to provide a balanced perspective on the magnitude of the risks, and also on the limitations of current knowledge. It would certainly be wrong to accept uncritically that all associations represent causal links, just as from another perspective sceptics, who in the face of mounting evidence, postulate ever more sources of bias and confounding and demand yet more definite proofs, may never be convinced. The conclusion from this section will be that passive smoking does pose a real threat, albeit one which is small by comparison with active smoking and hard to demonstrate unequivocally at the level of the individual. This provides the background for the remainder of the paper which considers how the issue has changed the nature of the

debate about smoking and gives examples of actions aimed at reducing this threat to public health.

Passive smoking as a cause of disease

Composition of mainstream and sidestream smoke

Non-smokers are exposed to the smoke given off by the smouldering tip of the cigarette between puffs (sidestream smoke), as well as to smoke which is inhaled by the smoker (mainstream smoke) and then breathed out again. Sidestream smoke forms about 80% of the total smoke. The chemical constituents of sidestream and mainstream smoke are essentially similar, although the relative concentrations of many compounds vary, reflecting the different combustion conditions during and between puffs. For example, tobacco-specific nitrosamines, which are powerful animal carcinogens, are found in 20 to 30 times the concentration in sidestream as in mainstream smoke. However, it would be wrong to assume that passive smokers could ever be more at risk than active smokers, for the good reason that, even discounting all the effects of active inhalation, those who smoke themselves are also the most heavily exposed passive smokers. Smoke from cigars and pipes is similar to that from cigarettes, and since tobacco smoke contains a number of known carcinogens, there are prima-facie reasons to suppose that it might be harmful to non-smokers' health.

How much are non-smokers exposed?

It might be anticipated that the risk to non-smokers' health should be in proportion to the dose they receive. Measurement of cotinine concentrations in blood, saliva or urine has provided a means of quantifying dose by comparison with active smokers. Cotinine is a major metabolite of exposure to tobacco smoke over the previous two or three days (Jarvis *et al.*, 1984). Studies on a range of population groups have shown that less than 10% of non-smokers have undetectable concentrations of cotinine and thus can be regarded as truly non-exposed. Cotinine levels bear a dose–response relation to self-reports of the extent of recent exposure, or to surrogate indicators such as spouse smoking. Figure 1 shows that saliva cotinine concentrations in non-smoking children are strongly influenced by their parents' smoking habits, with mothers' smoking having a greater effect than fathers'.

Children both of whose parents smoke take in on average about 1 to 1.5% of the nicotine intake of the 20 a day cigarette smoker, or the nicotine equivalent of themselves smoking 80 to 100 cigarettes each year. The most heavily

exposed non-smokers identified so far are people working in pubs and bars, whose exposure has been found to be equivalent to about half a cigarette's worth of nicotine each day.

Studies of this kind indicate that one cigarette's worth per day is likely to be close to the upper limit of non-smokers' nicotine uptake from passive smoking, even among those living continuously in heavily polluted atmospheres. The average exposure in the population will be much less. It might therefore be anticipated that non-smokers' risk of a variety of smoking-related diseases should be in similar proportion to this dose. Epidemiological studies are needed to determine whether exposure at these levels is in fact associated with measurable health consequences, although since there appears to be no threshold level of active smoking at which adverse effects are not detectable, even exposure at low levels would be expected to be harmful.

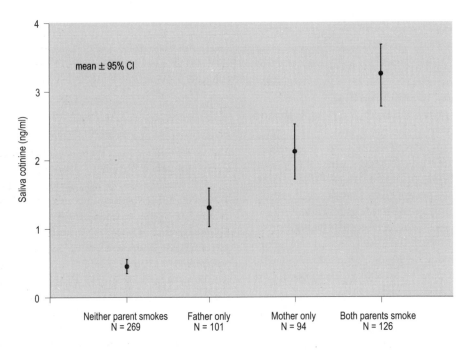

Figure 1 Saliva cotinine concentration in 569 non-smoking teenage schoolchildren by parental cigarette smoking habits. (Data are from Jarvis *et al.*, 1985)

Passive smoking and lung cancer

Of the approximately 40,000 deaths each year from lung cancer in the UK, some 3,000 are in non-smokers. Lung cancer is thus a rare disease among non-smokers, occurring at a rate of about 10 per 100,000 each year. Given this rarity, it is not easy to collect sufficient cases for scientific study. To date, some 24 published studies from different countries around the world have examined possible associations between passive smoking and lung cancer, evaluating the risk in non-smokers (mainly women) with smoking spouses with that found where both partners were non-smokers. These studies have been of two kinds: case-control, where index cases with lung cancer are compared with controls matched for age and other relevant variables but not suffering from lung cancer, and prospective cohort studies in which a sample of the population is followed over time until a sufficient number of non-smoking lung cancer cases has been accumulated to enable the investigation of possible associated factors. The single largest study was of a Japanese cohort initially recruited in the 1960s (Hirayama, 1981). A statistically significant increase in risk of lung cancer was found in wives whose husbands smoked, and there was evidence of a dose–response relationship, with a higher risk where the husband smoked more.

Considering these studies as a group, a clear trend emerges towards a positive association between lung cancer and having a smoking spouse. But in most cases the effect fails to reach statistical significance, reflecting partly the small sample sizes involved. A number of groups of independent scientists in the USA, Britain, Australia and elsewhere have carefully scrutinized the evidence (US National Research Council, 1986; National Health and Medical Council, 1986; Wald *et al.*, 1986; Fourth Report of the Independent Scientific Committee, 1988; Wald *et al.*, 1991). They have concluded that it is legitimate to pool findings to derive a more reliable estimate of the risk than can be obtained from the studies considered singly.

When this is done the observed increase in risk of lung cancer in non-smokers with smoking spouses is about 30% above that in non-exposed non-smokers.

Before accepting this link as causal, consideration has to be given to potential sources of bias. The main one that has been proposed is possible misclassification of smoking status (Lee, 1988). It is known that non-smokers tend to live with non-smokers and smokers with smokers (so-called aggregation of smoking). It is also likely that some individuals knowingly or through forgetting will say they have never smoked when they currently or used to smoke. This in conjunction with the aggregation of smoking habits could give rise to a spurious association, which would reflect concealed active smoking rather than passive smoking. While it is recognized that there is some force to this objection, it is unlikely to explain other than a small proportion of the observed increase in risk. Expert groups have concluded that the true increase in risk allowing for misclassification bias is in the range 10 to 30%. This translates into an extra 1 to 3 deaths per 100,000 non-smokers each year in the UK, or about 300 deaths annually. In the USA, a recent report from the Environmental Protection Agency has estimated a total of 3,800 lung cancer deaths in non-smokers each year attributable to passive smoking (US Environmental Protection Agency, 1990).

The evidence that passive smoking causes lung cancer has now been accepted by the British, US and Australian governments, among others. The case for accepting that passive smoking causes lung cancer rests on biological plausibility, consistency of association, magnitude of excess risk appropriate to known exposure levels, dose–response relationships, and lack of convincing alternative explanations. The remaining sceptics who seek more definitive evidence than that currently available before being convinced will probably never be satisfied given the intrinsic difficulties of studies in this area.

Passive smoking and disease in children

The first reports of health effects of passive smoking concerned babies and young children with smoking parents, who were found to be at greatly increased risk for admission to hospital with bronchitis and pneumonia (Colley *et al.*, 1974; Harlap and Davies, 1974). Subsequent research has established these effects beyond all reasonable doubt. Mothers' smoking has consistently been found to have a greater effect than fathers', reflecting their greater contact with their children. Studies from China, where 70% of men but very few women smoke, have replicated Western findings, indicating that apparent passive smoking effects cannot be attributed to later effects of mothers' prenatal smoking.

It has not been proved possible to explain the effects of parental smoking in terms of potential confounding variables such as social class or housing conditions. Nor would it appear that respiratory symptoms in children are due simply to cross-infection from parents themselves experiencing smoking-related respiratory conditions (this would be still be caused by parental smoking, but indirectly rather than directly through passive smoking).

A number of reports have shown associations between passive smoking and some impairment of lung function in children, and between passive smoking and glue ear (*otitis media*). A recent study on seven-year-olds from Edinburgh confirmed these observations and, by showing a direct link with exposure as quantified by saliva cotinine, provided strong evidence that the associations were causal (Strachan *et al.*, 1989; Strachan *et al.*, 1990).

The literature on passive smoking in children is highly consistent. It is not surprising that babies and young infants with delicate and developing respiratory systems should be most vulnerable to environmental smoke pollution. In terms of public health, the main burden of passive smoking almost certainly falls on children. A consequence of this in terms of regulatory measures is that passive smoking may be hardest to control where it has its greatest effects – in the home.

Cardiovascular effects of passive smoking

Heart disease provides a good example of the difficulties of reaching an unequivocal interpretation of passive smoking findings, and possible pitfalls. Twelve of 13 published studies have found evidence that passive smoking is associated with an increased risk of major coronary events, including death from ischaemic heart disease. The increase in risk, at about 25%, is of the same order as that for lung cancer in non-smokers with smoking spouses. Because heart disease is so common, an increased risk of this order would imply, if causal, a very large number of deaths. Indeed, recent estimates have suggested that passive smoking may cause some 37,000 deaths each year in the USA from cardiovascular disease out of a total of 50,000 passive smoking deaths (Glantz and Parmley, 1991). These estimates are reached on the basis that the entire increase in risk associated with exposure to passive smoking represents a causal effect.

There are strong reasons for caution in accepting this conclusion. There is no doubt about the association, but its interpretation as causal is open to question. In the first place, heart disease, unlike lung cancer which is almost entirely due to tobacco use, is multifactorial in its aetiology. Smoking is only one of the three major identified risk factors, the others being high blood pressure and high blood lipid levels. This immediately raises the possibility of confounding. It is known that smokers eat a more atherogenic diet than non-smokers. It is also highly likely that non-smokers living with smokers would tend to share their diet to some extent. This being the case, diet and passive smoking are confounded, and it is not possible to determine their relative contributions to the observed association.

A second reason for caution lies in the magnitude of the effects. The risk of heart disease in smokers is about double that in non-smokers (whereas their risk of lung cancer is 20 fold higher). An increase of 25% therefore represents a substantial proportion of the smoking risk, and seems inexplicably high in relation to non-smokers' dose from passive smoking, at 1% or less of active smokers' intake.

Summary of health effects

This has been a brief and selective review of some of the main health effects of passive smoking. No consideration has been given to what for many non-smokers is of most immediate concern – namely irritation of eyes, nose and throat. This is not to play down the significance of such proximal effects of tobacco smoke pollution, which do much to motivate non-smokers' desire for protection. However, it is undoubtedly the possibility that passive smoking causes serious disease and death which has fuelled the public debate. Equally, no mention has been made of asthma, lowered birth weight in babies, or sudden infant death syndrome. For each of these there is suggestive evidence, but which still has to be regarded as inconclusive, that passive smoking may play a part.

We are on firm ground in concluding that passive smoking does have a significant health impact. It is responsible for extensive respiratory disease in infancy and childhood and causes lung cancer in adult non-smokers. At the level of the individual, effects are hard to identify unequivocally, but because so many are exposed to tobacco smoke pollution, the public health burden is not inconsiderable. Lung cancer attributable to passive smoking by itself accounts for an estimated 300 deaths each year in Britain and the total number of passive smoking deaths must be considerably greater (Russell *et al.*, 1986). Sir Richard Doll, the distinguished epidemiologist, has estimated that the public health burden of passive smoking is more than an order of magnitude greater than that due to the operations of the nuclear industry worldwide, or of living and working long-term in asbestos-containing buildings. In both of these

areas regulatory authorities make great efforts to protect the individual.

The scope for action to clear the air

There is no doubt that the emergence of the passive smoking issue has changed in a fundamental way the debate about the public acceptability of smoking. An argument can be made that individuals have the right to engage in behaviours, however risky, when they knowingly undertake those risks and stand to harm only themselves. But when the well-being of others is threatened the rights issue is turned upside down. Clearly, the right of the non-smoking bystander to breathe in unpolluted air must take precedence over the right of smokers to enjoy their habit.

Two strands can be identified in the motives of those seeking to restrict non-smokers' exposure to other people's tobacco smoke. The first is obvious, and concerns elimination of the direct threat to non-smokers' health from passive smoking. The second is not usually stated but is of far greater scope. Passive smoking kills a few hundred people each year in Britain but active smoking causes 110,000 deaths. Increased restrictions on smoking in public places reflect a decisive shift towards lowered public acceptability of the smoking habit itself, and a major effect is to increase the desire of smokers to give up. The public health benefit may be more from reduced smoking-related disease in smokers induced to quit than from a lowered risk to non-smokers.

Thus a campaign against passive smoking is also a campaign against smoking itself. It is because the tobacco industry is well aware of this fact that it has devoted so much of its energies to combating this one issue.

Legislation

Legal restrictions on smoking in public places have been adopted in a number of countries in Europe and elsewhere. These include Ireland, Spain, Norway, the Netherlands, Belgium, Australia, Canada and the USA (Wald *et al.*,

1991). The extent of restrictions varies – for example, restaurants are included in Ireland but not Norway or Belgium. In the United States, which has been a leader in this area, much of the activity has been at the state level, but federal legislation now bans smoking on all domestic flights of up to six hours' duration.

Government in Britain has so far resisted any moves toward legislation, except in a few workplaces where controls operate on safety and hygiene grounds. Piecemeal activity at a local level has followed evidence of widespread public support for increased non-smoker protection (e.g. a survey by the European Commission in 1987 found that 72% of those questioned in the UK favoured a ban on smoking in public places). British Airways now operates smoke-free internal flights within the UK, but not on flights to Europe. London Transport took the opportunity offered by the Kings Cross disaster to introduce a ban on smoking throughout the underground system, and further restrictions on buses have followed. A complete ban on smoking on buses in Edinburgh came into effect in April 1991.

Arguments about the value of legislative approaches will no doubt continue. It is certainly true that a ban which lacks statutory support but which is effective is preferable to legislative gestures which are not enforced. Visitors to more than one European country will see within minutes of arrival at the airport that legal restrictions on smoking are totally ignored.

In its response to the recent House of Commons Environment Select Committee report on Indoor Pollution (Environment Committee, 1991), the government has accepted the need for stronger action. The Department of the Environment has announced that it is drawing up new guidelines which recognize that non-smoking should be the norm inside buildings and provides a code of good practice for segregation of smokers and non-smokers. This still falls short of actual legislation.

Legal test cases

Test cases brought to establish health effects of passive smoking are a powerful means to influence employers, since ignoring such judgements would lay them open to claims of compensation for personal injury. In Britain no case has yet succeeded in the law courts, but last year a woman won a ruling from the Social Security Commissioner that she had become incapacitated from working by her colleagues' smoking. Earlier this year an Australian judge ruled against the tobacco industry in a landmark case which evaluated the scientific evidence concerning passive smoking and lung cancer (Everingham and Woodward, 1991). This led state governments to prepare further legislation to ban smoking in all workplaces and employers to take anticipatory action.

Workplace smoking restrictions

The main environments in which non-smokers are exposed to tobacco smoke are the home and the workplace. It is much easier to introduce restrictions on smoking at work than it is to do anything about the home, and a great deal of activity on passive smoking has focussed on smoking at work. One reason for this is that employers are concerned about possible prosecution for breaching the Health and Safety at Work Act. Other considerations attractive to employers are reduced costs for cleaning and refurbishment, lower fire risk, and reductions in sick pay.

Some smokers faced with the introduction of restrictions on smoking at work have attempted to argue that this represents an unwarranted variation in the terms of their employment contract amounting to constructive dismissal. But there is no right to smoke. Although this is a matter which has to be handled sensitively and with due notice being given, there is no legal impediment to bringing in restrictions on smoking at work (Jenkins *et al.*, 1987). The Health Education Authority has published a useful guide to the important practical issues of how best to carry out consultation with the workforce, the most suitable type of policy and appropriate timescales. ASH now operates a consultancy service to help guide companies through the problems that can arise. So strong has the move towards workplace policies been that it is estimated that three out of every four of the top 500 British companies now operate a no-smoking policy. An Australian study which examined the acceptability and impact on smoking of a total workplace smoking ban at Telecom Australia found that by 18 months 81% of all staff, and 53% of smokers, approved of the ban. There were also measurable changes in smoking behaviour, with smokers consuming 3 to 4 cigarettes fewer per work day, and smoking prevalence declining by about double the rate in the community generally (Hocking *et al.*, 1991.

Smoking in the home

The home is rightly regarded as the last bastion of privacy, the one place that is safe from the tentacles of bureaucracy. Smokers who have worked all day in a no-smoking office and travelled home on no-smoking public transport are likely to reach for a cigarette as soon as they sink into their favourite armchair. No-one would wish to legislate away this freedom, but unfortunately the consequences for the non-smoking members of the family, particularly children, represent the major health impact of passive smoking. What can be done to reduce the effects of passive smoking in the home?

Many of the measures which have been discussed above have been at the level of government or of management, with a strictly limited role for the individual, other than as a concerned citizen. But it is arguable that health care professionals, especially those working in primary care, can have a valuable individual role in combating passive smoking through their daily contact with smokers. They can serve as sources of information and can advise on health-related behaviour. In both of these respects their contribution is respected and valued by the public. There is strong evidence

that simple advice from GPs given in the course of routine consultations is effective in inducing a small, but clinically worthwhile, proportion of smokers to quit (Russell *et al.*, 1979). Often, though, the majority who do not respond to advice are more salient than the few who do, and many primary care workers perceive themselves as concerned about smoking but ineffective in doing anything about it. What needs changing here is not the reality, since primary care intervention *is* effective (possibly the most effective intervention available at the public health level), but the self-perception.

Research which is currently underway is examining whether advice which specifically targets the passive smoking issue is a useful method of reaching parents with young children. Health Visitors see all mothers with newborn babies at a statutory post-natal visit. This may be a particularly receptive time for advice about passive smoking, since new parents naturally want to do all they can for their baby, and the newborn are especially vulnerable to the harmful effects of breathing in tobacco smoke.

Conclusion

In the past few years passive smoking has become the prime focus of smoking research and the central issue around which the public debate about smoking has revolved. It has transformed the argument about the right of individuals to harm themselves into a question of whether society can tolerate second-hand smoke harming others. The rights of non-smokers to be protected from tobacco smoke pollution have received increasing attention. The health effects of passive smoking are small by comparison with active smoking, but not negligible, and arguably greater than those of any other man-made environmental pollutant. We can expect to see moves towards increased restrictions on smoking in public places over the coming years, but ultimately reductions in passive smoking will depend on reducing the prevalence of tobacco smoking. The main health benefit will be not to non-smokers, but to those smokers who quit.

References

Colley, J.R.T., Holland, W.W. and Corkhill, R.T. (1974) Influence of passive smoking and parental phlegm on pneumonia and bronchitis in early childhood, *Lancet* **2**, 1031–1034.

Environment Committee (1991) Sixth Report, *Indoor pollution*, HMSO, London.

Everingham, R. and Woodward, S. (1991) *Tobacco legislation: the case against passive smoking*, Legal Books, Sydney.

Fourth Report of the Independent Scientific Committee on Smoking and Health (1988) HMSO, London.

Glantz, S.A. and Parmley, W.W. (1991) Passive smoking and heart disease: epidemiology, physiology and biochemistry, *Circulation* **83**, 1–12.

Harlap, S. and Davies, A.M. (1974) Infant admisions to hospital and maternal smoking, *Lancet* **1**, 529–532.

Hirayama, T. (1981) Non-smoking wives of heavy smokers have a higher risk of lung cancer, *Brit. Med. J.* **282**, 183–185.

Hocking, B., Borland, R., Owen, N. and Kemp, G. (1991) A total ban on workplace smoking is acceptable and effective, *J. Occupational Med.* **33**, 163–167.

Howard, G. (1990) Some legal issues relating to passive smoking at the workplace, *Brit. J. Addiction* **85**, 873–882.

Jarvis, M.J., Russell, M.A.H., Feyerabend, C., Eiser, J.R., Morgan, M., Gammage, P. and Gray, E.M. (1985) Passive exposure to tobacco smoke: saliva cotinine concentrations in a representative population sample of non-smoking school children, *Brit. Med. J.* **291**, 929–929.

Jarvis, M.J., Tunstall-Pedoe, H., Feyerabend, C., Vesey, C. and Saloojee, Y. (1984) Biochemical markers of smoke absorption and self-reported exposure to passive smoking, *J. Epidemiol. and Comm. Hlth.* **38**, 335–339.

Jenkins, M., McEwen, J., Moreton, W.J. *et al.* (1987) *Smoking policies at work*, Health Education Authority, London.

Lee, P.N. (1988) *Misclassification of smoking habits and passive smoking*, Springer-Verlag, Berlin.

National Health and Medical Research Council (1986) *Effects of passive smoking on health*, Australia.

Russell, M.A.H., Jarvis, M.J. and West, R.J. (1986) Use of urinary nicotine concentrations to estimate exposure and mortality from passive smoking in non-smokers, *Brit. J. Addiction*, **81**, 275–281.

Russell, M.A.H., Wilson, C., Taylor, C. and Baker, C.D. (1979) Effect of general practitioners' advice against smoking, *Brit. Med. J.* **2**, 231–235.

Strachan, D.P., Jarvis, M.J. and Feyerabend, C. (1989) Passive smoking, salivary cotinine concentrations, and middle ear effusion in seven-year-old children, *Brit. Med. J.*, **298**, 1549–1552.

Strachan, D.P., Jarvis, M.J. and Feyerabend, C. (1990) The relationship of salivary cotinine to respiratory symptoms, spirometry and exercise-induced bronchospasm in seven-year-old children, *Am. Rev. Respiratory Disease* **142**, 147–151.

Tobacco Advisory Council (1989) *Smoke and the non-smoker*, Tobacco Advisory Council, London.

Tobacco Advisory Council (1989) *Smoke and the non-smoker: scientific aspects of environmental tobacco smoke*, Tobacco Advisory Council, London.

Trichopoulos, D., Kalandidi, A., Sparros, L. and MacMahon, B. (1981) Lung cancer and passive smoking, *Int. J. Cancer* **27**, 1–4.

US Department of Health and Human Services (1986) *The health consequences of involuntary smoking: a report of the Surgeon General*, U.S. Department of Health and Human Services, Washington DC.

US Environmental Protection Agency (1990) *Health effects of passive smoking: assessment of lung cancer in adults and respiratory disorders in children*, Office of Health and Environmental Assessment, EPA.

US National Research Council Committee on Passive Smoking (1986) *Environmental tobacco smoke: measuring exposures and assessing health effects*, National Academy Press, Washington DC.

Wald, N.J., Booth, C., Doll, R. *et al.* (eds.) (1991) *Passive smoking: a health hazard*, Imperial Cancer Research Fund and Cancer Research Campaign, London.

Wald, N.J., Nanchahal, K., Thompson, S.G. and Cuckle, H.S. (1986) Does breathing other people's tobacco smoke cause lung cancer?, *Brit. Med. J.* **293**, 1217–1222.

HELPING INDIVIDUALS MANAGE THEIR RISK OF CANCERS

INTRODUCTION

The papers in the first two parts of this book have focussed on the ways in which data from a variety of disciplines and countries can build up a picture of the patterns of common cancers and the potential for preventing cancers. In the light of this, the challenge for health professionals is to find ways of working with individuals and with whole communities that actively change these patterns and bring about a reduction in mortality and morbidity from those cancers. The two final parts of this book start to address this challenge. Part 3 examines the ways in which health professionals can approach their work with individuals.

Beliefs and risk

In thinking about helping people to change their health behaviours it is important for health professionals to be aware of, and sensitive to, lay perceptions of disease and the way that individual people perceive the risks in their lives. Angela Hall points out in her paper 'Lay health beliefs about the causes of cancer', that health professionals and the people with whom they work may have very different views of the nature and causes of cancers. If these differences are not recognized, the chances of health professionals being effective in helping people to change their risk-related behaviour is reduced. Hall's paper draws on detailed published research into lay beliefs about the causes of cancers and the ways that ordinary people believe that cancers might be prevented. The conclusion is that individual people have a wide range of ideas and attitudes which health professionals need to understand. They should adapt their

health education approaches to suit the needs of the individual people whom they are in contact with and try not to make assumptions about people's health beliefs.

There is no such thing as a life free of risk. As individuals, we decide for ourselves what risks we are prepared to take and what risks we try to avoid. The task for health professionals undertaking preventive work is to help people make informed decisions about what risks they are prepared to live with and which behaviours they might wish to modify. It is the health professional's task to bring information about the size of particular risks related to cancers to people who approach them for help and to assist the people themselves to chose which options to take. Michael Henderson, in 'Risk and cancer', discusses the concept of risk and how it is assessed and perceived. Both individuals and the societies in which they live must manage risks and take responsibility for the consequences of doing so.

Helping individuals change to health enhancing behaviours

Many different factors influence the behaviours that people adopt in relation to their health, for example when deciding what to eat and drink or whether to smoke tobacco. The complexity of the reasons for these decisions, and the ways in which changes towards more healthy options can be brought about are examined by James Prochaska. In the paper 'What causes people to change from unhealthy to health enhancing behaviour?', Prochaska critically examines the concept of behavioural change. He suggests that unfocussed, diffuse health promotion programmes are unlikely to be successful in bringing about change. More specific programmes are required which are sensitive to the complex stages of behavioural change and which pay attention to causal factors that can be brought under the control of the individuals who are trying to change. Self-efficacy is an important concept discussed in the paper; this involves individuals who want to change particular health-related behaviours, maintaining a sense that they are in control and have the power to change within themselves.

Putting prevention into practice

Tobacco smoking is recognized as being the most dangerous and potentially the most preventable carcinogenic activity, causing at least one-third of all cancers throughout Europe. The majority of people who decide whether to smoke or not have usually taken this decision during childhood and have already formed their habit by the time they are young adults. It is quite unusual for people to take up the smoking habit after their mid-twenties. Childhood and adolescence are the times to influence people's smoking behaviour for life. Tobacco companies recognize this and make efforts to attract youngsters to the habit in order to replenish the size of their market of older people who are killed by tobacco, or who decide to give it up. The best way to prevent tobacco-related cancers is to help young people not to start smoking.

In 'Young people and their smoking behaviour', Hein de Vries *et al.* draw particularly on the Dutch experience of health education focussed on young people. They outline the constituents of effective health education programmes with people of this age group and emphasize the importance of careful planning and evaluation of such interventions. Health education efforts should be based on a knowledge of the determinants of a particular behaviour. In the case of smoking in young people, these are attitudes, social influences, expectations of self-efficacy, psychological characteristics such as risk-taking or rebelliousness, and barriers such as the price and availability of cigarettes. School-based health education programmes can be formulated which attempt to tackle these factors. These programmes are more effective if they are supported by wider, community-oriented anti-smoking activities such as public information programmes, smoking cessation programmes and social legislation to increase the price and restrict advertising and sales of tobacco.

Early detection of cancers can play a further part in reducing mortality from cancers throughout Europe, but the value of particular interventions always needs to be critically examined. In their paper 'Breast self-examination', Joan Austoker and Julie Evans consider the place of breast self-examination (BSE) aimed at early detection of breast tumours. Because the precise causes of breast cancer are not yet determined and advances in the treatment of breast cancer have yielded only modest improvements in survival, early detection offers the best hope at present of improving death rates from breast cancers. In general, the earlier a breast cancer is detected, the better the survival prospects for that individual woman. Unfortunately, as Austoker and Evans point out, the promotion of BSE as a primary screening procedure is of unproven benefit and should be regarded as an intervention which may have a beneficial but limited effect.

3.1

LAY BELIEFS ABOUT THE CAUSES OF CANCER

Angela Hall

Doctors tend to hold illness representations based on biomedical conceptualizations of pathology; these are often mechanistic in nature. By contrast, lay representations of illness are likely to be more diverse and less firmly held. They tend to incorporate folk knowledge, as well as medical knowledge derived from personal experience and media sources. These are assumptions that are so embedded in both doctors' and patients' beliefs about the causes of illness that they may be unaware that they are not universally held.

The differences in these beliefs, and the assumption that each party shares similar beliefs, can give rise to considerable problems in communication. There can be disadvantageous consequences for the exchange of information, for decision making about treatment and for adherence to treatment and medical advice. The doctor–patient relationship as a whole may be adversely affected if the salient beliefs of the patient are ignored or discounted. This may add significantly to the burden of distress suffered by patients with chronic and/or life-threatening disease.

For most people, being given a diagnosis of cancer is tantamount to being handed a death sentence. Of those population surveys that have been carried out in the last twenty-five years, cancer is perceived with more alarm and considered more serious than any other disease. Knopf (1976) published findings of a survey conducted in 1973 compared with a baseline survey in 1966. Cancer was ranked first on a cumulative scale of five diseases assessing the alarm each provoked: over half of the sample in both surveys selected it as the single most alarming disease. There was a small increase in optimism: only 21% in 1973 thought it 'never curable', compared with 27%

in 1966. In both surveys, nearly two-thirds of the women thought cancer the major cause of death.

In fact, in 1973, including all types of cancer, there was a five-year recurrence-free survival rate of 47%. Cancer seems almost benign in comparison with stroke, where 50% of all patients died within a year, and myocardial infarction where 35% of all coronary patients were dead within a month of their heart attack (1973 figures).

The sparseness of research raises problems in forming a coherent understanding of lay explanations for cancer.

A literature search reveals some research whose focus is oblique to the specific topic of causal explanations for cancer, but which nonetheless has some relevant findings for it. One example is a study by Peters-Golden (1982) of 100 women with breast cancer and 100 disease-free women. The aim of the study was to examine perceived social support in the cancer patients and anticipated social support in the well individuals. Much evidence is cited to support the idea that cancer is a stigmatized condition, though a lot of it is from journalistic sources. However, it includes a quote from a study by Wortman and Dunkel-Schetter (1979) who claim that there is evidence that 'individuals are motivated to believe in a "just world" in which people "get what they deserve and deserve what they get". Since having cancer is such an undesirable fate, individuals may be strongly motivated to protect themselves by attributing the disease to others' undesirable personal characteristics or their past behaviour.' Presumably, then, 'blaming the victim' contributes to the imputation of stigma.

This study found that 56% of the healthy women said they would avoid contact with someone they knew who had cancer. In contrast, 72% of the breast cancer patients reported that they were treated differently after people knew they had cancer: 52% found that they were 'avoided' or 'feared', 14% felt they were pitied. Only 3% thought people were 'nicer' to them than previously. However, the authors appear to interpret those findings as evidence for the attribution of contagion, without considering the possibility that others may find the experience of approaching the patient too distressing to contemplate.

Some evidence for knocks or damage as a causal explanation can be found in a study by Fallowfield *et al.* (1990) which looked at the psychological factors influencing attendance for breast-screening. Thirty-five per cent of their sample of 122 women cited this type of trauma as making it more likely for a woman to develop breast cancer. However, this section of their questionnaire was concerned with knowledge about risk factors (e.g. parity, age, menopausal status) rather than lay beliefs. As such it did not allow for exploration of other possibilities such as stress, contagion, etc. More recent work (Rutter and Calnan; 1987, Payne, 1990) demonstrates the pervasiveness of this particular explanation.

One of the classic studies on ideas about disease causation was carried out by Blaxter (1983), who interviewed 46 middle-aged women of social classes IV and V. An unstructured ethnomedical approach was used, in which 1–2 hour conversations took place in the general context of health and illness. The women themselves chose which diseases they would talk about, and a verbal and content analysis was imposed to derive models of the structure of their linking. An interesting finding was that although cancer and tuberculosis were two of the diseases most frequently mentioned, they were also the most frequently mentioned without discussion of cause. Cancer was seen as the natural successor to tuberculosis and cited almost universally as the disease to be dreaded nowadays, but few women talked about it at

length. Of those who did consider cause, two thought that it was hereditary, a few suggested environmental agents and several thought that it could be brought on by something else such as an accident, an ulcer or fibrosis. Interestingly, the women rejected any firm connection between smoking and lung cancer. Blaxter states that:

> The women gave the impression of *preferring* to believe that cancer was quite randomly caused: 'it could happen to anyone'. But while they firmly rejected any idea of responsibility, part of the tenor of the disease was simply that it was mysterious … It seems possible that the relative lack of discussion about the cause of cancer, given its salience as judged by the number of times the disease was mentioned, was due not only to the fact that they believed the cause to be unknown (a fact which did not deter discussion of many other diseases), but also to a specific reluctance to talk about it. Cancer was … a condition to which a superstitious dread adhered, as well as a rationale and understandable fear – to talk about it was to invoke it, to speak briefly or in a lowered voice was to leave it sleeping.

Very similar results were obtained by Verres (1990), using semi-structured interviews with 101 healthy individuals in southern Germany. Twenty-five per cent declared spontaneously during the interview that fear of cancer could be a risk factor for cancer. 'They believed that talking as little as possible about cancer prevented them from going "crazy" and from becoming prone to cancer themselves.' The main question explored was whether subjective theories on cancer treatment are significant for the decisions people make about cancer treatment and for early detection of cancer. As such, the study was more concerned with knowledge of, and attitudes towards, cancer than with causal attributions and their role in decision making. However, Verres comes up with some fascinating results with implications for the medical profession and health educators.

There were two findings that may shed some light on how cancer sufferers themselves develop certain types of causal explanations for their disease. First, although 81% of the sample estimated that the general risk for human beings of getting cancer was quite high or very high, only 24% estimated their *own* risk at these levels. Forty-nine per cent said that they usually repress their own fear of cancer. 'This means that they tend to change the topic when conversations focus on cancer issues.' Thus, strong defences operate in people. Cancer patients experiencing these ambivalences and defences from others may well feel isolated and stigmatized, which may generate beliefs about contagion or punishment/retribution. In addition, the second finding could certainly contribute towards the formation of beliefs about contagion. The healthy respondents seldom admitted directly that they were afraid that cancer was contagious. However, asked about concrete behaviours referring to differing degrees of intimacy with cancer patients, a different picture emerged. Eighteen per cent stated that they would not want to eat something that a cancer patient had cooked, 32% would not want to drink from a glass that a cancer patient had used before and 42% expressed resentment about direct physical contact with cancer patients in intimate situations. Faced with these kinds of behaviour, a cancer patient cannot fail to feel, at the very least, unclean, if not downright infectious.

Linn *et al.* (1982) studied 120 patients with late stage cancer (mixed site) and compared them with non-cancer patients matched for age, sex and hospitalization. Beliefs about causes of cancer were measured at interview with a 10-item scale covering smoking, drinking alcohol, diet, inheritance, type of occupation, stress, medicine, water, environment, God's will and

'other'. The primary finding was that cancer patients held significantly less firm convictions about causative factors in the aetiology of the disease than did non-cancer patients. This differential held even for beliefs about smoking in patients with lung cancer. For cancer patients, 'God's will' and 'inheritance' were listed in the top four priorities for aetiology and there was a trend for cancer patients to endorse 'inherited' more if they had had the diagnosis of cancer for longer time. The authors point out that:

> It is common for patients told of terminal illness to feel confused and bewildered by their condition. The search for a reason, then, becomes much more personal. The person without cancer can afford to be more dogmatic about causes and likely to think in stereotypes. The closer he comes to dealing with the disease, the less clear-cut and more complex the explanations may become.

One study that focused squarely on causal attributions and their relationship to beliefs about control and adjustment was carried out by Taylor *et al.* (1984) on a sample of 79 American women with different stages of breast cancer. The authors point out that:

> Attribution theory … maintains that when one encounters a sudden threat or change in one's environment, one will initiate a causal search in an effort to understand that threat or change … Attributional search is thought to be initiated so as to understand, predict and control threat and hence may be especially functional early on in the adjustment process.

There were two hypotheses – first, that patients would make attributions for their cancer, and second, that attributions would be made early in the adjustment process, around the time of diagnosis. Hence, this study is unusual in that it specifies not only testable hypotheses but measurable outcomes. Ninety-five per cent of the sample, during long semi-structured interviews employing open-ended questions, revealed that they made causal attributions. In addition, a comparison group of significant others was asked whether *they* had any causal attribution for the patient's cancer. Sixty-three per cent of them had – a difference significant at the .01 level 'suggesting that the need for an explanation is greater among patients'. However, the prediction that attributions would be made early on in the adjustment process was not supported.

Taylor *et al.* then considered the *content* of respondent's attributions. Stress (41%) was most frequently cited, followed by a specific carcinogen (32%), heredity (26%), diet (17%), blow specific to the breast (10%) and other (28%). Twenty-four per cent of the sample held theories involving two or more causes. Interestingly, no one theory or belief was better for adjustment than any other. Looking more specifically at responsibility attributions, which presumably included causes mentioned under 'other', the researchers found that 41% of the sample blamed themselves, 10% blamed another person, 28% blamed the environment and 49% blamed chance. However, whether blame was assessed at interview or on questionnaire responses, no simple relation was found between self-blame and adjustment. Moreover, looking at self-blame may be adaptive at some times and not others. Only blame of another person (usually one's physician or (ex-) spouse) was significantly related to poor adjustment, associated with unresolved anger and distress.

Cook Gotay (1985) claimed that no study to date had addressed the existential question, 'Why me?', and set out to assess responses both to this question and to specified kinds of possible causes. She was also interested in whether different causal attributions predominate at different stages in the disease process. She interviewed 42 women with early stage cervical cancer and 31 women with advanced stage gynaecological or breast

cancer. 'Why you?' was asked as an open-ended question, while the possible causal attributions fell into four categories: 'Yourself – the kind of person you are', 'Things you have done', 'The environment and other people' and 'Chance'. The partners of 10 early stage and 20 advanced stage patients were also interviewed and asked the same questions, in relation to the patient.

Between one-fifth and one-quarter of all respondents reported that they had not asked themselves 'Why me?'. Fourteen per cent of early stage and 26% of advanced stage patients had asked themselves the question, but failed to come up with an answer. With the exception of advanced stage patients, both patients and partners were most likely to feel that it was chance. Interestingly, the patients were most likely to cite religiously-based reasons, '… God has a reason and I have to accept it as that'. It is worth noting that 14% of early-stage women cited 'past behaviour', presumably reflecting the much documented association between early sexual activity and multiple partners in the development of cervical cancer. Most other causes, such as inheritance, personality etc., were mentioned only by very small percentages of patients and their partners. Turning to the fixed categories, the largest proportion of blame in all groups was allocated to chance. However, advanced stage patients and their partners were significantly more likely to attribute the development of cancer to the individual herself. Things that the patient had done were given significantly more weight by patients than by their partners, who gave more consideration to chance factors.

A well-known study by Pill and Stott (1985), which focussed on beliefs, attitudes and practices in the area of preventative health behaviour in healthy women, also revealed that the majority of their respondents were to some degree fatalistic about health and illness. They did not find evidence of cognitive strain, however, among the many women who perceived health and illness as a matter of chance, but who also had some degree of belief in the importance of lifestyle decisions for health and who had developed more complex views which could embrace both concepts. Although the authors were particularly interested in the implications of this finding for health educators, one conclusion may also be relevant to Cook Gotay's findings:

> What, from one point of view, may be seen as 'fatalism' may, from another perspective, be interpreted as a realistic appraisal of the complex variables involved in the aetiology of illness ... an appraisal rooted in actual experience and constantly reinforced through interaction with others from the same background.

In a study of 269 women with early breast cancer, first reported by Fallowfield et al. (1990), preliminary analysis of data on causal attributions has shown that many women asked themselves the question 'Why me?', but failed to come up with any definite answer. However, a considerable number inverted the question, to ask 'Why not me?', indicating a belief in the random nature of its attack. Among the remaining women, 'trauma to the breast' or 'stress' were more commonly cited, though not necessarily as unicausal factors. It was not uncommon for women to view themselves as being at risk in some way through, for example, the operation of hereditary factors or because 'we all have cancer cells within us', with the development of their tumour being triggered by more specific factors. Many women who felt that stress was the proximate cause of their cancer emphasized their wish to change the stressful aspects of their lives, which they hoped would prevent the onset of recurrence and give a feeling of having some control over the course of their disease. A small number of women viewed the development of their cancer as retribution for past 'sins'.

The stories of retribution were among the most powerful that were related to the interviewers, and the women themselves amongst the most distressed. Interestingly, there was no suggestion that getting cancer atoned for these 'sins'; this is an area that merits further research.

Kroode et al. compared the causal attributions of 33 mixed-site cancer patients with those of 14 patients following myocardial infarction. Data were collected in long, unstructured interviews. The study was concerned with identifying sources of conflict between patients' idiosyncratic views and medical opinion. In contrast to the previous study, Kroode et al. found that nearly all of the patients, regardless of diagnosis, had thought about the cause of their illness. However, substantial differences appeared between patient groups in terms of their causal attributions. Myocardial infarction patients were found to go through and check their autobiographies, looking for possible causes suggested by the medical world. Cancer patients on the contrary searched for possible explanations with 'idiosyncratic, very personal attributions with which they create an explanation which is often not in accordance with the physician's view'. Thus, most cancer patients had two accounts – the formal, medical one and the informal, idiosyncratic one. Myocardial infarction patients formed only one – an informed medical explanation. The authors feel that this difference is explained by the dreadful negative associations, both literal and metaphorical, of cancer. Cancer patients feel victimized by their disease in a way unknown to patients with heart disease. In fact, the latter group talked with some pride about hard work and consequent psychological stress, even though they saw these life habits as unhealthy. The other explanation, not surprisingly, stems from the lack of scientific knowledge about the cause and course of most types of cancer. If doctors cannot give cancer patients a satisfactory explanation for their illness, then the patients are thrown back upon common sense models and their own imagination.

Three areas of conflict were identified in the cancer patients. First, an internal conflict generated by ambivalence between the formal medical and the idiosyncratic explanations: 'They are caught between belief and disbelief and therefore subject to an internal conflict'. Myocardial infarction patients also doubted whether the known risk factors for an infarction held in their own case, but these doubts did not give rise to this kind of internal conflict. Second, conflict with the physician arose out of the clash between idiosyncratic beliefs and unsure aetiological beliefs. Nearly half of the cancer patients had never talked about their causal attributions with anyone else, which probably indicated that they anticipated this conflict and wished to avoid it. Certainly those patients who did talk to their physician about their personal explanations were not satisfied with their reception, which was largely dismissive. Third, discussion about cause was also withheld from nearest relations. This, of course, was due at times to the patients' wish to avoid a conflict with those whom they felt had had a direct part to play in causing the illness in the first place. In addition, though, cancer patients thought that their relatives would take the physician's side, supporting the formal, medical view and rejecting the personal beliefs of the patients. The authors conclude that 'in spite of these three conflicts, the cancer patients keep to their own stories, be it often secretly and with ambivalence. Apparently they are very important to them'. Although the sample was small, this type of in-depth approach is very important as a means of disentangling the strands that contribute to cancer sufferers' explanatory frameworks and understanding their significance.

References

Blaxter, M. (1983) The causes of disease: women talking, *Soc. Sci. Med.* **17**(2), 59–69.

Cook Gotay, C. (1985) Why me? Attributions and adjustment by cancer patients and their mates at two stages in the disease process, *Soc. Sci. Med.*, **20**(8):825–831.

Fallowfield, L.J., Rodway, A. and Baum, M. (1990) What are the psychological factors influencing attendance, non-attendance and re-attendance at a breast screening centre?, *JRSM* **83**, 547–551.

Fitzpatrick, R. (1984) Lay concepts of illness. In Fitzpatrick, R., Hinton, J., Newman, S., Scrambler, R. and Thompson, J. (eds) *The experience of illness*, Tavistock Publications.

Knopf, A. (1976) Changes in women's opinions about cancer, *Soc. Sci. Med.* **10**, 191–195.

Kroode, H.T., Oosterwijk, M. and Steverink, N. (1989) Three conflicts as a result of causal attributions, *Soc. Sci. Med.* **28**(1), 93–97.

Linn, M.W., Linn, B.S. and Stein, S.R. (1982) Beliefs about causes of cancer in cancer patients, *Soc. Sci. Med.* **16**, 835–839.

Payer, L. (1989) *Medicine and culture*, Victor Gollanz Ltd.

Payne, S. (1990) Lay representations of breast cancer, *Psychol. and Health* **5**(1), 1–12.

Peters-Golden, H. (1982) Breast cancer: Varied perceptions of social support in the illness experience, *Soc. Sci. Med.*, **16**, 483–91.

Pill, R. and Stott, N.C.H. (1985) Choice or chance: Further evidence on illness and responsibility for health, *Soc. Sci. Med.* **20**(10), 981–991.

Rutter, D.R. and Calnan, M. (1987) Do health beliefs predict health behaviour? In Dent, H. (ed.) *Clinical psychology: research and developments*, Croom Helm, New York.

Sontag, S. (1978) *Illness as Metaphor*, McGraw-Hill Ryerson Ltd., Toronto.

Stoeckle, J.D. and Barsky, A.J. (1981) Attributions: Uses of social science knowledge in the 'doctoring' of primary care. In Eisenberg, L. and Kleisman, A. (eds) *The relevance of social science for medicine*, D. Reidel Publishing Co, 223–240.

Taylor, S.E., Lichtman, R.R. and Wood, J.V. (1984) Attributions, beliefs about control and adjustment to breast cancer, *J. Personality Soc. Psychol.* **46**(3), 489–502.

Verres, R. (1988) Subjective theories in etiology and treatment of cancer. In Scheurlen, H., Kay, R. and Baum, M. (eds) *Recent results in cancer research. Cancer clinical trials: a critical appraisal*, Springer-Verlag, London.

Wortman, C. and Dunkel-Schetter, C. (1979) Interpersonal relationships and cancer, *J. Soc. Iss.* **35**, 120.

RISK AND CANCER

Michael Henderson

Concepts of risk

> The proper function of man is to live, not exist. I shall not waste my days in trying to prolong them. I shall use my time.

Jack London, who wrote these words, was not suicidal. But in 'using his time' he went adventuring in a way that to many people showed a reckless disregard of risk. Yet those same critics every day made personal judgements on what to them were, or were not, acceptable risks.

We all must die, nearly all of us within 95 years or so of our birth, and that total life span has not extended much since Biblical times. The big change in the developed world has been the huge increase in the proportion of us who survive childhood and live through a healthy middle age.

It is in making the most of these middle years of life that we make all those choices, and all those decisions, which aim to minimize the chance – the 'risk' – of premature death and illness, while maximizing our enjoyment of life.

Thus, every day we take some risks and avoid others. In few cases do we assess risk in a truly objective manner. We accept the need for a chest X-ray, as well as its carcinogenic risk, because it is recommended by a doctor, or because we feel more comfortable about ourselves if it shows no abnormality. Similarly, we drive to work, or take the bus for that matter, because the benefits of so doing seem to us easily to outweigh the risk of crashing. But when it comes to cancer, what little objectivity most of us have in living with risk becomes overwhelmed by our perceptions and prejudices.

People are scared of cancer, despite the preventability and treatability of many kinds of it. But we cannot all avoid it, any more than we can avoid many other hazards. We cannot reduce the risk of it to zero, any more than other risks can be reduced to zero. There is no such thing as absolute safety, the complete absence of risk, even though some of our actions, our writings, and our demands on administrators appear to imply that zero risk is a realistic aim (Slovic, 1987).

We turn therefore to 'assessment' of risk in order to give some expression – usually numerical – to degrees of uncertainty.

Assessment of risk

Risk and uncertainty

When data are lacking, assessments become highly subjective. To help us make sound assessment and choices, we need information. Sometimes that information comes to us through trial and error, sometimes we have to seek it out. If, on the one hand, we wrongly perceive a high risk when the real risk is low, we may miss out on substantial benefits. On the other hand, we may wrongly perceive that some activities carry a far lower risk than they really do. If we think that smoking can do little harm, we are more likely to choose to smoke. If we think our driving is faultless, why put our child in a safety seat?

The science of risk assessment is rapidly emerging as a sensible way of examining risks so that they may be better avoided, reduced, or otherwise managed. Risk assessment, except in the most simple of cases, does not make decisions for us. It illuminates the decisions that we make.

When risks have been with us for a long time, we can use historical data to measure them. They are then easy to understand, and are often perceived quite accurately.

For risks of cancer, however, all calculations are complicated by the long delay between exposure to the hazard and the onset of the disease (Wilson and Crouch, 1990). For conditions with a high incidence and epidemiological data, cancer from cigarette smoking, for example, it may be possible to put reliable, hard figures on risks to humans. But when historical data are lacking, and the actual risk small, we have to turn to analogy, usually by looking for cancer risks to animals.

To translate data obtained this way involves some difficult translation: the carcinogenic potential of a substance may be very different for animals and humans. For example, it proved hard to show that tobacco smoke was carcinogenic in rats, yet it is powerfully so in humans. If a chemical is carcinogenic for rats but not mice (or vice versa), it is quite possible that it is not carcinogenic for man. Dioxin definitely causes cancer in rats; but whether it does so in humans is unclear.

It is hard to extrapolate from the short-term high doses of suspicious substances that are given to animals, to the low doses over a longer term that humans might encounter (Fishbein, 1980).

Then there is the question of uncertainty.

The concepts of risk and of uncertainty are closely related. The lifetime risk of cancer may be 25%, meaning that about 25% of us will develop it. But once an individual does develop cancer, the concept of 'risk' disappears because there is no longer any uncertainty. With a high degree of certainty we know that vinyl chloride causes angiosarcoma in both rats and humans. When very few people are exposed, the total number of occurrences is very small and the risk to populations is very small. On the other hand, we think – while being far from certain – that saccharin may carry a small risk of cancer for

humans. Nevertheless, hundreds of thousands of people are exposed to it. Thus, the risk to total populations is higher, although there is much more uncertainty about the value of the risk. Some would concentrate their attention on vinyl chloride in this situation, some on saccharin. There is no 'right' or 'wrong' way of looking at risks.

Comparisons of risk

Comparisons of risk can be useful for putting some meaning into magnitude, preferably when the methods of measurement are the same: comparing travel by bus and by car, for example.

Another example is the use of animal tests in the prediction of cancer risk among humans. These tests cannot be used to predict absolute human risks. They can, however, be used to indicate that some chemicals may be of greater concern than others. Bruce Ames, in a comprehensive and most valuable review (Ames et al., 1987) has ranked possible hazards to humans presented by a variety of rodent carcinogens by an index that relates the potency of each carcinogen in rodents to the exposure in humans. Such a ranking suggests that carcinogenic hazards from current levels of synthetic chemicals in the environment are of minimal concern in comparison with the background carcinogenic effect of natural substances, and he gives several provocative examples to highlight what many will see as a paradox.

For example, plants produce 'natural' pesticides to protect themselves against insects and fungi, and moulds synthesize a variety of toxins as antibiotics in the microbiological struggle for survival. We consume in our diet at least 10,000 times more by weight of these natural pesticides than man-made pesticide residues. Yet few that have been tested are in fact carcinogenic. Nitropyrenes in diesel exhaust have been shown to be carcinogenic too, but intake of these nitropyrenes is hundreds of times higher from eating burnt food than it is in the most polluted street. One of the most potent carcinogens for rats is over-eating, but how often do we discuss obesity as a human carcinogen? New synthetic food additives are screened for carcinogenicity, yet we do not question the use of alcohol, a known carcinogen, as an additive.

The point is not that we should be constantly worrying about 'natural' carcinogens, but that we should keep concerns about 'synthetic' carcinogens in perspective. There is no point in pursuing hundreds of minor or doubtful hazards while ignoring the really important carcinogens, such as tobacco.

Comparisons can also heighten the drama of contrasts. Take the carcinogenic effects of aflatoxin and dioxin, for example. In animal species, they both have a potent carcinogenic effect. However, whereas there is a high degree of *certainty* about the carcinogenicity of aflatoxin, there is less certainty about dioxin, especially in man. Nevertheless, the two chemicals are treated quite differently in the community. Aflatoxin is permitted in foodstuffs at low levels. Yet even the smallest trace of dioxin, if found, say, in ground water, becomes a matter for vigorous environmental concern and public calls for action.

Why is dioxin seen as so much more dreadful? This question brings us to the very different ways in which risks are perceived.

The perception of risk

Once a risk has been identified, a decision has to be made as to whether to do anything about it, and if so, what. In democratic societies, several groups are involved in such decisions: the public and community groups, political parties, and experts and managers. In an ideal world, experts gather scientific evidence and give technical advice to the politicians, who then legislate and regulate for the benefit of, and with the implicit agreement of, the community.

In practice, of course, things do not work out that way. A high potential for mistrust and

misunderstanding lies in the fact that people, whether within groups or as individuals, see things differently from each other. One of the things they see – 'perceive' – differently is risk.

When the world was a less complex place, without media to disseminate fearful information, there was less scope for differences in perception of risk. At the individual level, the hazards faced by ordinary people were accepted and coped with daily: fire, water, cold, heights and so on. The risks to worry about were the risks one faced oneself.

The really big change is that as part of the process of technological evolution, 'new' hazards have emerged, posing risks that individuals might know about, but that do not affect them directly and cannot be controlled. As viewed through the pages of the tabloids and the screen of a television, the world can look like a very dangerous place (Henderson, 1990).

Mental manipulations

To make sense out of complicated issues, such as their evaluation of risk, people use a set of strategies that in the jargon of psychology are called 'heuristics' (Kahneman *et al.*, 1982). These rules of judgement can lead to perfectly valid and reliable assessments, but sometimes to substantial bias and to disagreement with people who have used different patterns of thought to evaluate the same set of facts.

The mental trick with perhaps the most significant implications for the perception of risk is the 'availability' heuristic, whereby the situation under review is matched with information that is most readily available and easily recalled. Thus, the more 'available' the information on a given event, the more likely it is judged that the event will occur. Things which really do often happen are, of course, easy to bring to mind, but there are many other factors that influence recall. These include the regular and repeated reporting of events that are truly not very frequent, and exposure to dramatic information that is rich in death and disaster. In this way, the more unusual and dramatic (and often fatal) happenings are likely to be perceived as more frequent than they really are.

This proposition has been tested by several research workers. A pioneering team in Oregon (Lichtenstein *et al.*, 1978) started this line of enquiry by asking rather different groups of people to judge the frequency of various causes of death. Their studies showed that while judgements were moderately accurate, in the sense that people generally knew what were the most frequent and least frequent lethal events, there were still several seriously wrong judgements and these seemed to reflect bias that was consistent with the 'availability' hypothesis. Most of the frequent hazards did elicit higher estimates. However, there was a clear tendency among participants to overestimate the incidence of rare causes of death and underestimate the frequency of the common ones.

An important potential effect of the availability heuristic is that people may not easily be assured by frequent reiteration of the fact that a rare event will rarely happen. A safety engineer may wish to show the rarity of a disaster by stressing the number of safety features built into a nuclear power plant. However, if he does so by repeated detailed descriptions of them, the result may be the perception that the supposedly rare event is, in fact, rather likely, as 'proved' by the number of safety features that are needed to prevent it.

What makes a risk look 'risky'

Examination of the ways in which various groups evaluate risk shows that while experts use statistics and fatality rates to assess and rank them, other people do not. They must, therefore, be using another set of concepts and beliefs to do so. A British group, having performed a set of studies very similar to those performed in Oregon, has concluded that it is the *qualitative* aspect of risk that is important in determining perceptions, rather than the *quantitative* (Green and Brown, 1978).

Clearly then, perception of risk is a much more complicated matter than the use of statistics would indicate, and depends very much on personal biases and the context in which the risk is introduced into society. Thus, mental images are drafted that help to determine the perceptions. The use of nuclear power, it can be argued, is associated with images of nuclear bombs and mushroom clouds, and thus with the possibility of the types of nuclear explosions at power plants that experts maintain are impossible. Imagine that petrol, an extremely common source of energy used daily by almost everyone, had been introduced into public perception through its use as napalm or as a powerful explosive (which it is). Perceptions of the risk associated with carrying the stuff around in a metal tank in the family car could well, thereby, have been very considerably different from what they are now.

Our perception of risk depends a great deal on how the facts are presented.

Public policies on the management of risk will be threatened if they challenge values and opinions that are firmly held, especially when the risk is perceived as being of a potentially catastrophic nature. Formal, 'technical' presentations of risk are of rather little value. The problem is not that 'objective' characterizations of risk and the statistical calculations that accompany them are more correct or more real or more valid than the subjective assessments of risk performed by the majority of the population. It is simply that they are *different*, and represent the fact that the world is seen in different ways by different people.

The 'technologists', including 'experts', are comfortable with the use of numbers, and believe that the world and its systems are under human control and management. On the other hand, there are those who believe that feelings are more important than numbers, that the world's systems are delicately balanced, and should not be upset by human intervention.

The acceptability of risk

In this paper the words 'safe' and 'safety' have been avoided, because they imply a zero-risk situation that for practical purposes cannot be attained. In choosing between activities with different levels of risk or in managing a given situation so that risk is to be minimized, what we are working towards is a level of risk that is 'acceptable'. It is the level that most people will regard as 'safe', or at any rate 'safe enough' (Schwing and Albers, 1980).

This is not to say that they are necessarily happy about it. Everyone will prefer less risk to more risk if the benefits stay the same. The trouble is, each successive reduction in risk achieves a bit less and costs a little more, such as when reducing the levels of trace carcinogens in drinking water (National Research Council, 1986).

How safe is safe enough?

Judgement that a risk is acceptable is not something that depends (for most people) on numbers, but is more usually a subjective determination using value judgements. People in one locality will violently oppose the burying of low-level nuclear waste in their vicinity, despite expert assurances of safety, while people living under high dams in earthquake areas happily ignore expert warnings of disaster. Some would have it that it is impossible to define a 'negligible' risk in numerical terms. Mathematical analysis of probabilities can be used to prove to an individual that the risk of contracting cancer from the water supply is, say, one in a million over the next 50 years, but the actual question he wants answered is, 'Is the water safe or will it give me cancer?'

In the case of public administration of risks affecting whole communities, people are inherently suspicious of what is done – or not done – on their behalf. Measurement has shown that what people are prepared to accept under these circumstances is a level of risk that is very much lower than the level of

risk that they accept voluntarily. For these situations, and for the circumstances faced by a worker in a hazardous environment, there is a big difference between a risk that is acceptable and a risk that must be accepted.

At this point, what people will then regard as 'safe enough' depends a great deal on the confidence that they have in the way that risks are managed, and it is to management that we now turn.

Management of risk

The management of risk is a matter of day-to-day decision-making for us all. At the personal level, managing risk does not necessarily mean reducing it. The skier who flies to Switzerland for a fortnight on the slopes is choosing not to *minimize* personal risk, but rather to face it and embrace it as part of an attempt to maximize the enjoyment and quality of life.

At the level of public administration, risk management is the process of deciding what to do in cases where risks have been determined to exist. An 'acceptable' risk is the risk associated with the best of the *available* alternatives, not the best alternative we can think of. Thus, managing risk means integrating risk assessment with feasibility and economic reality.

As part of any such process, several different groups will be involved, and examples of the ways that such groups may disagree have already been touched upon. Arguments on risk reduction – improvements in safety – are likely to centre on the *feasibility* of introducing the necessary measures, their *cost* and their *inconvenience*.

Different countries have different ways of expressing their aims in legislation. With respect to industrial safety, for example, in Norway and Sweden there is an implicit assumption that safety depends on the environment rather than the worker. In the United Kingdom (where the employer is enjoined to ensure 'so far as is reasonably practical' the health and safety of his employees) and in the United States ('... as far as possible ...') there is a feeling that we can legislate to move towards a goal but not to require its attainment (Singleton, 1987).

Public participation is increasingly part of risk management in large utilities, especially where the production of power is concerned. Participation may be formal, as in public enquiries, or informal, as through the pressure of public opinion expressed in the media. Participation also raises the risk of confrontation between politicians, public, experts and managers. Lawyers become involved, raising the black-or-white issues of the courts. And all competing groups will differ on the importance to be placed on technical evidence.

Just as a great advantage of risk assessment is bringing calculations out into the open, uncertainties and all, so one of the great advantages of risk management has been bringing the decision process out into the open.

Education therefore plays a fundamental part in risk reduction. People may reach their conclusions on an entirely different basis from that used by technologists. When information genuinely is inadequate and experiences biased, education may help to bridge the gap. As part of the process of policy determination, people's knowledge and attitudes can be studied to deduce ways in which such gaps in understanding can best be narrowed. The sharing of knowledge more widely does not ensure that decisions will reach universal approval. But when ignorance prevails, the extent of disagreement and disapproval will almost inevitably be greater.

Further, people must believe that risks are being accurately reported to them, especially in the case of 'dread' events of very low probability but potentially catastrophic consequence. The trick is to build that public confidence. There is some evidence that where the safety of consumer products is concerned,

formal analysis of risk is preferred as a basis for making decisions over the informal practices that, in general, represent the standard industry approach today.

Management in practice

The actual techniques employed for managing risk at the societal level include the following (Pease, *et al.*, 1990):

- avoiding or eliminating the risk, such as prohibiting the use of a potentially dangerous substance or activity;

- regulating the use of the substance or activity to reduce adverse health effects, such as defining what food additives are permitted and controlling the sale of chemicals;

- reducing the vulnerability of people and property, such as by requiring the use of forced ventilation or protective clothing;

- developing mitigation and recovery procedures after the event, such as the establishment of rescue units and specialized medical teams;

- instituting schemes to reimburse and redistribute losses, such as insurance and extra pay for high-risk jobs.

Public acceptance of a risk does not mean that people find that risk acceptable. So, for the purpose of management, it is convenient to divide risks into three groups:

- events of very high risk and unacceptable consequences;

- events of very low risk with negligible consequences;

- risks falling between those two extremes that require management for maximum benefit.

Some risks are so high that managers and decision-makers can reasonably expect that nearly all individuals would find the risk unacceptable. A continuing risk of death of one in 100 each year, imposed over and above risks existing from all other sources, is essentially too high to be publicly acceptable. The more dangerous voluntary sports and activities, such as those of professional stuntmen, approach this sort of level, and some exceed it.

Several review bodies have speculated that few people would commit their resources to reduce an annual risk of death that was already as low as one in 10,000 and even fewer would take action at an annual level of one in a million. A one-in-a-million risk is about the same as that from dying from a prescribed drug or a vaccination, or of a meteorite killing a thousand people, or of an aeroplane crashing into an empty football stadium around London, and it is lower than the risk of dying from an earthquake in California. A chemical with a one-in-a-million risk of causing cancer would kill 50 people in Britain in 70 years (a lifetime), or less than one a year.

There is of course a big difference between a one-in-a-million chance of killing a million people in a given year, and the chance of one person a year dying every year for a million years. Public perceptions of these two outcomes of the same risk are very different. In practice, the risk of a disaster that is prominent in the public mind (such as the catastrophic disruption of a nuclear reactor) has to be reduced to somewhat below what, for other less 'dread' events, would be regarded as acceptably low levels.

The limits within which risks should most appropriately be managed, therefore, embrace a range of between about one in a thousand and one in a million.

Costs and benefits

A few already tiny risks may be reduced even further at very low cost, but inevitably at some point there will be reached a situation where to reduce risk further would need unjustifiable expenditure. It follows that a necessary part of risk management is to take account of benefits and in some way balance them against the risks that are being reduced.

Perhaps the most intractable problem is that, because many risks of public interest are most effectively measured in terms of death or, at best, reduction in life expectancy, some monetary value has to be placed, for comparative purposes, on human existence. Further, at that point it is very easy for the discussion to become distorted. For example, the question 'How much should we spend per life saved?' is very different from the question that many people take to be an inevitable corollary, namely, 'How much is a life worth?' It is not necessary to answer the second question to cope with the first.

Cost-benefit analysis is always liable to moderation on a case-by-case approach, with the importance of the individual generally paramount. Imagine that a huge foodstore required fumigation to prevent the growth of a mould that could result in the death from cancer, over the next 20 years, of (say) a dozen people. However, the necessary fumigant chemical (for which there was no alternative) was hazardous to the workers to the extent that one or two would be likely to die – also from cancer – within this period. It is unlikely that such a fumigant would be permitted although its use would represent a net community gain, because the near certain death of one or two people in a small group is regarded generally as a matter of much greater concern than the possible death of more people but among a very large number.

In a situation where outlays are necessarily limited, resources are best devoted to those risks in which the most reduction is achieved for every pound expended. There are, nevertheless, some consequences that are so horrendous that extraordinary measures will be justified in reducing the risks, however small or vague they are. For example, chlorofluorocarbon aerosol impellers (CFCs) may be destroying ozone in the stratosphere, and thus potentially upsetting the earth's entire temperature balance. If they do, it will be too late to do anything about it afterwards. There are alternatives. So, most governments are moving towards a ban on them.

Risk and responsibility

All groups in society bear some responsibility for the effects of public decisions on risks. Individuals or pressure groups who succeed in getting a pesticide banned globally can take credit for any reduction in cancer deaths but will also be responsible for any extra deaths that might occur, such as through increases in mosquito-borne disease for example. If coal-burning power stations are used to replace nuclear power stations because of the risk of cancer through radioactive contamination, and if this results in an exaggeration of the 'greenhouse effect' on the world through the continuing release of carbon dioxide, then those responsible for the decision are also responsible for the potentially catastrophic environmental changes that could occur as a result. None of this makes lobbying 'right' or 'wrong'. It is just that we must realize that any decision on risk is a decision that affects us all.

The role of the professional health care worker is to ensure that people – as communities, families and individuals – gain a greater understanding of how risks are measured, represented and managed. The aim is to help people make rational choices. It makes no sense for an individual who smokes to demonstrate about a supposedly carcinogenic food additive. It makes no sense to worry about little risks and ignore the big ones.

Health workers concerned with the management of risk can present choices to people in such a way that they are helped to understand the balance that exists between risks and benefits, and how risk management can paradoxically make things seem more dangerous than they are. Well understood substances with well known effects – good and bad – are not more 'risky' simply because we know what the real risks are. There is no such thing as zero risk. Those who constantly seek it may force the use of substances and systems which in fact present a greater threat. Because we do not know about a risk does not mean it is not there. A new substance is not necessarily better than an old; a natural substance is not necessarily better than a synthetic one.

We live in a complicated world. We all must realise that if we assign our priorities in managing risks so that resources are *not* distributed in a maximally effective manner, then the result is that people will die before their time, and those premature deaths could have been prevented.

References

Ames, B.N., Magaw, R. and Gold, L.S. (1987) Ranking possible carcinogenic hazards, *Science* **236**, 271–280.

Fishbein, L. (1980) Overview of some aspects of quantitative risk assessment, *Journal of Toxicology and Environmental Health* **6**, 1275–1296.

Green, C.H. and Brown, R.A. (1978) Counting lives, *J. of Occupational Accidents* **2**, 55.

Henderson, M. (1990) *Living With Risk*, Penguin Books, London.

Kahneman, D. *et al.* (eds.) (1982) *Judgement under uncertainties: heuristics and biases*, Cambridge University Press, New York.

Lichtenstein, S. *et al.* (1978) Judged frequency of lethal events, *J. of Experi. Psychol.: Human Learning and Memory* **4**, 551.

National Research Council (1986) *Drinking water and health*, National Academy Press, Washington, DC.

Pease, W.S., Zeise, L. and Kelter, A. (1990) Risk assessment for carcinogens under California's Proposition 65, *Risk Analysis* **10**, 255–271.

Schwing, R. and Albers, N. (eds.) (1980) *Societal risk assessment: how safe is safe enough?*, Plenum Press, New York.

Singleton, W.T. (1987) Risk handling by institutions. In Singleton, W.T. and Horden, J. (eds.) *Risk and decisions*, John Wiley and Sons, New York and Chichester.

Slovic P. (1987) Perception of risk, *Science* **236**, 280–285.

Wilson, R., and Crouch E.A.C. (1990) Risk assessment and comparisons: an introduction, *Science* **236**, 267–270.

WHAT CAUSES PEOPLE TO CHANGE FROM UNHEALTHY TO HEALTH-ENHANCING BEHAVIOUR?

James O. Prochaska

To address this question intelligently requires that we first define what we mean by *change*. After all, behavioural change is the goal that unites professionals in the field of health promotion and disease prevention. One of the factors that has retarded the field is our traditional reliance on a relatively unsophisticated concept of change. Most often we have implicitly defined change as the movement from chronic unhealthy behaviour to stable healthier behaviour. Change was seen as a dramatic shift from one stable but less healthy state to another stable but healthier state. An example of such dramatic shifts is smokers going from smoking 20 cigarettes a day for 20 years to no cigarettes a day for the next 20 years.

What is wrong with this conceptualization, besides the fact that it does not represent the way that most people change? First of all, it leads us to expect people to change quickly. So we offer short-term smoking cessation programmes that last from four to six sessions, and we are disappointed that 70 to 80% of the participants are still smoking a year later (Hunt and Bespalec, 1974). Or we offer 12 to 24 session weight-control clinics and we are distressed that 70 to 80% of the participants are still obese between 12 and 24 months later (Stunkard, 1977).

People do not change chronic behaviours quickly. The best data that we have available indicate that average self-changers take three to four serious 'quit' attempts spaced out over seven to 10 years before they successfully quit smoking (Prochaska and DiClemente, 1984; Schacter, 1982). And we expect to be successful with one trial of intervention spaced out over seven to 10 weeks? We have been treating chronic behaviour problems as if they were acute disorders.

The traditional conceptualization leads us to expect change to be a dichotomous event. People should shift from eating unhealthy diets to healthy diets, from being smokers to non-smokers, from sedentary lives to active lives and from fat to trim. People do not change chronic behaviours discretely. It is much too simple-minded to divide up clinic participants into discrete categories such as smokers and non-smokers. It is also very expensive to use discrete categories for intervention research. In the smoking area, for example, we are stuck with the standard of counting the proportion of smokers and non-smokers as our ultimate outcome criteria. Tests of proportions have such limited power that we are forced to have samples of hundreds or thousands to detect significant effects of our interventions. If we could rely on more continuous outcome measures we could use much more powerful statistics that could reduce our research expenses to just a fraction of the 1 to 3 million dollars required for a smoking cessation study.

Alternative concepts of change

Let us examine an alternative conceptualization of change that may do more justice to how people change and our attempts to help people change. In retrospective, cross-sectional and longitudinal studies of self-change, and in intervention studies we have found that change involves movement through a series of stages (DiClemente and Prochaska, 1982; Prochaska and DiClemente, 1983; Prochaska, DiClemente, Velicer, Ginpil and Norcross, 1985). Initially we identified four stages: precontemplation, contemplation, action and maintenance.

Precontemplation is a stage in which people are not seriously thinking about change, at least not in the next 6 months. We use a 6-month criterion because that seems to be about as far out in time as people seriously plan health behaviour changes. Contemplation is the period during which people are seriously thinking about changing an unhealthy behaviour in the next 6 months. Action is the 6-month period following an overt modification of an unhealthy behaviour.

Initially we compared 0 to 3-month periods and 3 to 6-month periods and found no differences in the action strategies people use to continue to quit smoking. So we grouped these people together into a 0- to 6-month action stage (Prochaska and DiClemente, 1983). Maintenance is the period from 6 months after an overt behaviour change until the problem behaviour is finally terminated. Termination we define as zero temptation across all problem situations and maximum confidence in one's ability to resist relapse across all problem situations. Maintenance is a period of continued change, while termination is a much more stable state.

We can measure these stages discretely using a simple 5-item algorithm or continuously using a 32-item questionnaire (McConnaughy, Prochaska and Velicer, 1983). We can make finer discriminations in the stages, such as contemplators who are ready for action, which includes people who have relapsed in the past year and are thinking seriously about taking action in the next month. What happens when we classify people into different stages of change rather than dichotomize them into smokers and non-smokers? Figure 1 presents the percentage of smokers in different stages who took action during the first six months of an intervention study. Figure 1 includes approximately 570 smokers from four different self-help interventions.

Figure 1 indicates that approximately twice as many smokers in the contemplation stage took action as those in the precontemplation stage. Similarly, nearly twice as many contemplators ready for action quit for at least 24 hours than did the contemplator group. To treat all of these smokers as if they are the same would be ludicrous. And yet, that is what we traditionally have done in our dichotomous definition of change.

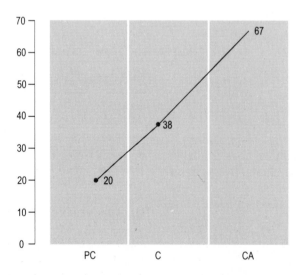

Figure 1   Per cent taking action by 6 months of smokers who were in the precontemplation (PC), contemplation (C) and ready-for-action (CA) stages prior to intervention

In an intervention study with smokers with heart disease, Ockene (1989) and other colleagues found that 22% of the smokers who were in the precontemplation stage prior to treatment were not smoking at a 6-month follow-up. Of those who were in the contemplation stage, 44% were not smoking at 6 months, and approximately 80% of those ready for action or in action were not smoking at 6 months. So, even with people with life-threatening heart diseases, there is a doubling of smoking cessation between precontemplators and contemplators and between contemplators and those ready for action or in action at the start of the study.

Compared to our relatively healthy sample of smokers, three times as many patients with heart disease were not smoking at 6-month follow-up. Furthermore, patients with 50% or more blockage in three arteries quit at significantly higher rates than those with blockage in one artery. These data suggest that behaviour change is a function of (a) health status, (b) severity of disease and (c) stage of change independent of health status.

Our traditional prevention programmes have implicitly assumed that our prospective participants are ready to take action on their unhealthy behaviours. We design state-of-the-art action-oriented programmes and then are disappointed by how few people participate in our programmes. Schoenbach, Orleans and Wagner (1988) surveyed a representative sample of smokers in a Seattle HMO and found that 70 to 80% said they would take advantage of a self-help smoking cessation programme if it were offered for free. The HMO then offered a state-of-the-art nicotine fading action-oriented programme with considerable publicity and fanfare. They were disappointed when only 4% of the smokers signed up over a 6-month period.

David Abrams and his colleagues did a similar survey for a work site self-help programme (Abrams, Follick and Biener, 1988). Knowing the disappointing sign-up rate for the HMO study, Abrams and his colleagues used behavioural incentive principles to encourage people to sign up. They offered opportunities to win prizes and days off from work just for signing up. They increased the sign-up rate dramatically from 4% to 7%.

Timing interventions

The vast majority of our prevention programmes are designed for the small minority of the people who are ready to take action on their health behaviour problems. Using the best data we have available from a national survey, we can estimate what percentage is in each stage at any one time (USDHHS, in press). Of those individuals who were smoking in 1985, at what stage were they in 1986? These estimates indicate that 4% were in the maintenance stage, 12% were in action, 15% were ready for action, 34% in contemplation and 35% in the precontemplation stage.

Even with a health behaviour problem that has received the most publicity, has the greatest consensus about its deleterious consequences, and has 10 million people served by NCI intervention research projects alone, nearly 70% of the smokers are not ready to take action on their smoking. In a recent survey in Seattle, 62% of the respondents said they weren't even thinking about changing their diets in order to reduce their fat intake (Deborah Bowen, personal communication).

We must stop pretending that all we have to do is deliver state-of-the-art action programmes to the people and they will take advantage of them. We must shift our national research agenda from diffusing weaker and weaker health promotion programmes to more and more people who are not prepared to use them.

If we are to better serve the majority of people with health behaviour problems, such as smoking, obesity, inactivity and high-fat diets, then we need to address such questions as: What causes people to begin to think seriously about changing unhealthy behaviours? What

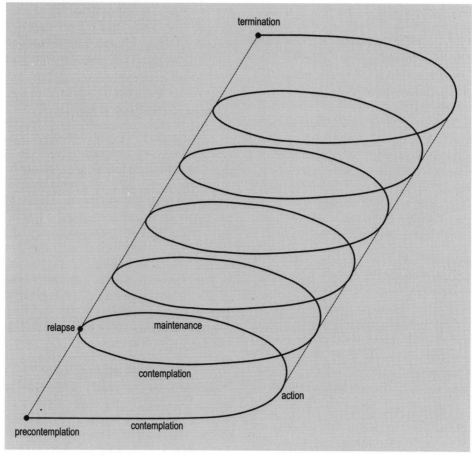

Figure 2 Progressing to the tower of change

causes chronic contemplators to eventually become ready for action? What causes those in action to struggle to keep from relapsing? What causes nearly 85% of smokers who relapse to recycle back to contemplation rather than give up on themselves? And what causes people to eventually maintain their change activities until they finally terminate their temptation to relapse?

There is nothing in the stages of change model that suggests that precontemplators will automatically, dramatically, and discretely progress to the next stage of change. As a matter of fact, we found that of the nearly 200 precontemplators we followed every 6 months for 2 years, approximately two-thirds remained in the precontemplation stage the entire time (Prochaska, DiClemente, Velicer, Rossi and Guadagnoli, 1989).

Learning from relapses

A spiral model more adequately represents how the majority of people change over time. Figure 2 illustrates how people with chronic behaviour problems progress from precontemplation to contemplation to action. The majority relapses on any one cycle through the stages. Fortunately, the vast majority of those who relapse do not give up on themselves, but rather recycle back to the contemplation stage as they prepare for further action. The spiral pattern suggests that most people learn from their relapse experiences rather than going in circles.

Our current work on causal modelling suggests that different factors cause people to move from precontemplation to contemplation than cause people to progress from contemplation to action; in prospective studies, for example, we used 17 subject characteristics to try to predict progress from one stage to the next. These included age, education and income, smoking history, reasons for smoking, previous quit attempts, withdrawal symptoms, health history including presence of life-threatening diseases and intensity of positive and negative life changes in the past 6 months. Two of these variables, smoking for pleasure and smoking over a long period, predicted remaining in the contemplation stage.

For relapses, however, higher income and education and fewer daily cigarettes predicted continuing to move ahead following a relapse. None of the 17 variables predicted progress for either contemplation to action or action to maintenance.

Predicting progress between stages

In a comparison study we found that 14 dynamic process variables served as much better predictors of progress from one stage to the next than did the more static subject and problem characteristic variables (Prochaska *et al.*, 1985). With the contemplators, for example, those individuals who progressed to action were initially higher on the cons of smoking, self-efficacy, and self re-evaluation; and lower on consciousness raising, the pros of smoking and temptations to smoke. From our prospective studies to date, we have concluded that it is not who you are or who you know that counts, but what you do and when you do it.

We have also concluded that different variables produce progress at different stages of changing unhealthy behaviours. Working from a related stage model, Rosen and Shipley (1983) concluded that different sets of

variables predict changes at each stage of change.

In a worksite-based behavioural weight control study, the challenge was to predict both attendance and outcome for those who signed up for the action-oriented programme (Prochaska, Norcross, Abrams and Fowler, 1989). Abrams and his colleagues had found in three different worksites that approximately 80% of those who enrolled in the programme dropped out. We used the best predictor variables we could find, including demographics, problem history, health history, goals and expectations, self-efficacy, social support for changing, and the stages and processes of change.

The stages of change was the second best predictor of outcome. The more subjects who were in the action stage early in treatment, the more weight they lost at follow-up. The single best predictor of change for both attendance and outcome was the processes of change that participants were using early in treatment. The dynamic processes of change outperformed such important but static variables as socio-economic status, percentage overweight, years overweight, family weight history, and social support for attendance and weight loss. The behavioural weight control programme was fine for participants who were ready for action but was failing those who were not.

What causes people to change?

In trying to answer the global question of what causes people to change to healthier behaviours, we are likely to find that more static variables such as age, education, income, gender, race, and health status predict global changes from smoker to non-smoker, unhealthy diet to healthy diet or sedentary to more active lifestyles (e.g. USDHHS, 1989). The problem with these causal variables is that they are imposed on people rather than being under the control of people. Age, socio-economic status, gender, race and health status are imposed on us for the most part rather than determined by us. At a minimum, these causal factors are not under the potential control of professionals trying to facilitate change. Nor are they under the immediate control of the individuals who are needing to change.

In trying to answer more specific questions, such as what causes people to move from contemplation to action, we fortunately are likely to find that more dynamic variables, such as decisional balance, self-efficacy and processes of change, determine specific changes from one stage to the next. The advantage of these causal variables is that they can be immediately controlled by people rather than imposed on people. At a maximum, these causal factors can be brought under the potential control of professionals trying to facilitate change. And these causal factors can be under the immediate self-control of the individuals who are needing to change.

References

Abrams, D.B., Follick, J.J., and Beiner, L. (1988, November) *Individual versus group self-help smoking cessation at the workplace. Initial impact and twelve month outcomes.* In T. Glynn (Chair) Four National Cancer Institute-funded self-help smoking cessation trials: interim results and emerging patterns. Symposium conducted at the Annual Association for the Advancement of Behaviour Therapy Convention, New York.

DiClemente, C.C., and Prochaska, J.O. (1982) Self-change and therapy change of smoking behaviour: a comparison of processes of change in cessation and maintenance, *Addictive Behaviours* **7**, 133–142.

Hunt, S.A. and Bespalec, D.A. (1974) An evaluation of current methods of modifying smoking behaviour, *J. Clin. Psychol.* **30**, 431–438.

McConnaughy, E.A., Prochaska, J.O and Velicer, W.F. (1983) Stage of change in psychotherapy: measurement and sample profiles, *Psychotherapy: theory, research and practice.*

Ockene, J. et al. (1989) *Smoking cessation in cardiac patients: the coronary artery smoking intervention study.* Manuscript submitted for publication.

Prochaska, J.O. and DiClemente, C.C. (1983) Stages and processes of self-change in smoking: toward an integrative model of change, *J. of Consulting and Clin. Psychol.* **5**, 390–395.

Prochaska, J.O. and DiClemente, C.C. (1984) *The transtheoretical approach: crossing traditional boundaries of therapy*, Dow Jones/Irwin, Homewood, Illinois.

Prochaska, J.O., DiClemente, C.C., Velicer, W.F., Ginpil, S. and Norcross, J.C. (1985) Predicting change in smoking status for self-changers, *Addictive Behaviours* **10**, 395–405.

Prochaska, J.O., DiClemente, C.C., Velicer, W.F., Rossi, J.S. and Guadagnoli, E. (1989) *Patterns of change in smoking cessation: between variable comparison.* Manuscript submitted for publication.

Prochaska, J.O., Norcross, J.C., Abrams, D.S. and Fowler, J. (1989) *Attendance and outcome in a worksite weight control programme. Processes and stages of change as process and predictor variables.* Manuscript submitted for publication.

Rosen, T.J. and Shipley, R.H. (1983) A stage analysis of self-initiated smoking reductions, *Addictive Behaviours* **8**, 263–272.

Schacter, S. (1982) Recidivism and self cure of smoking and obesity, *Am. Psychol.* **37**, 436–444.

Schoenbach, V.J., Orleans, C.T. and Wagner, E.H. (1988) *Recruiting smokers to a self-help cessation study in an HMO: the free and clear experience.* Unpublished manuscript, School of Public Health, University of North Carolina at Chapel Hill, Chapel Hill, NC 27514.

Stunkard, A.J. (1977) Behavioural treatment for obesity: failure to maintain weight loss. In Stuart, R.B. (ed.), *Behavioural self-control*, Brunner/Mazel, New York.

US Department of Health and Human Services (in press) *Adult use of tobacco, 1986*. US Department of Health and Human Services, Public Health Services, Centres for Disease Control, Office on Smoking and Health.

US Department of Health and Human Services (1989) *Reducing the health consequences of smoking: a report of the Surgeon General*. US Department of Health and Human Services, Public Health Services, Centres for Disease Control, Centre for Health Promotion and Education, Office on Smoking and Health.

YOUNG PEOPLE AND THEIR SMOKING BEHAVIOUR

Hein de Vries, Margo Dijkstra and Gerjo Kok

Introduction

Many people take up smoking during adolescence. When health professionals stressed the dangers of smoking to health, the assumption was that these messages would enhance youngsters' negative attitudes towards smoking, and thus prevent the uptake of smoking (Thompson, 1978). The effects of these programmes were mostly limited to an increase in knowledge, and did not have significant effects on behaviour (Leventhal and Cleary, 1980). The main reason for this limited effect is that smoking is determined by several motives. This has been clearly recognized by tobacco companies as their campaigns often connect several positive consequences with smoking, such as adulthood, increased attractiveness, etc. During the last decades, however, smoking prevention interventions that focussed on several determinants have been more successful. In discussing the various strategies we will first describe a health promotion planning model, and then focus in more detail on the major determinants of smoking, the various intervention strategies and the strategies for diffusion.

Planning interventions

The effectiveness of interventions is dependent on careful planning and evaluation of the intervention (Green and Kok, 1990). The ABC Health Promotion Planning model based on insights of Green et al., (1980), de Vries and Kok (1989) and Rogers (1983) distinguishes three phases (see Figure 1).

Analysis of the problem

During this phase, several issues are analysed, such as the severity of the health problem, its relation to human behaviour, the behavioural determinants and their preventability, and the target groups.

Behavioural change

A central theme in this phase is the development, pre-testing and evaluation of an intervention. A choice of intervention strategy has to be made. Two main types of strategies are feasible: *health education activities*, such as school programmes, out-of-school activities, a community approach and public information campaigns; and *legislative activities*, such as reducing the availability of cigarettes and making smoking prevention mandatory at schools. We will focus here mainly on the health education activities. An intervention has to focus on the relevant determinants and has to be pre-tested to detect negative side effects. Finally, evaluation is necessary to analyse whether the implementation was implemented as planned (formative evaluation), attractive and appealing (programme evaluation), and whether it successfully changed the determinants and behaviour (effect evaluation).

Diffusion of a successful programme requires diffusion strategies, supportive health policies, and a broad intersectoral health promotion approach.

A: ANALYSIS OF THE PROBLEM

  1 Is the problem serious?

  2 Which behaviours?

  3 Which determinants?

  4 Which target group?

B: BEHAVIOURAL INTERVENTION

  1 Choice for intervention strategy

  2 Development of intervention

  3 Evaluation of intervention

C: CONTINUED PREVENTION

  1 Diffusion strategies

  2 Health promotion policies

  3 Intersectoral approach

Figure 1   The ABC Health Promotion Planning Model

Determinants of smoking

Smoking is the result of an interplay of various different factors (see Figure 2).

Attitude

The attitude of an adolescent is dependent on a variety of factors connected with smoking (Ajzen and Fishbein, 1980). These include the knowledge of the health risks, personal disadvantages (e.g. expense) and the personal and social advantages (e.g. acceptance by peer group).

Social influences

Adolescent smoking behaviour is also influenced by the norms and behaviour of important people from their social environment. The impact can be exerted directly via persuasion (Evans *et al.*, 1978), slightly less directly via norms of others (Ajzen and Fishbein, 1980), and indirectly via the perception of behaviour of others which may stimulate imitation (Bandura, 1986).

Self-efficacy expectations

Self-efficacy refers to a person's expectation about their ability to perform a specific behaviour. Adolescents have to feel confident about their skills to remain a non-smoker. For instance, a non-smoker has to feel able to resist peer group pressure.

Psychological characteristics

Smoking behaviour is also related to specific characteristics such as rebelliousness, risk-taking and sensation-seeking. Self-esteem and academic values may mediate the effects of the social environment. The impact of these factors is probably indirect via the attitudinal, social and efficacy factors.

Barriers

Smoking onset is also related to factors determining the availability of cigarettes, especially the price and accessibility of purchase.

Behavioural interventions: school-based prevention programmes

During the last decades, several successful smoking prevention studies have been developed (Best *et al.*, 1988; Tobler, 1986), and recently recommendations for smoking prevention research have been documented by Glynn (1989) and the UICC (1990). The major factors determining the effectiveness of these programmes are: (a) the content, length, educational technique, participants, provider, setting and the context.

A smoking prevention programme should at least cover information on (a) the short and long-term health and social consequences of smoking and the advantages of non-smoking; (b) the social influence process which affects smoking; (c) modelling and skills training to resist pressure to smoke and a discussion of the alternatives to smoking (de Vries, 1990;

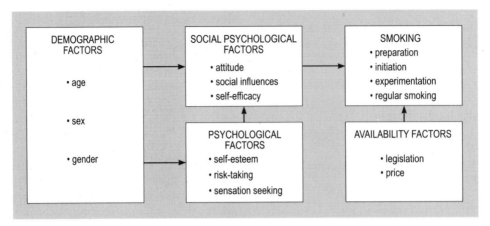

Figure 2   Model of the determinants of smoking

Glynn, 1989; UICC, 1990). A minimum of 10 classroom sessions is recommended (Glynn, 1989). The educational techniques should include group discussions and active learning principles to stimulate involvement and intake of information, and the use of videos and manuals to enhance the programme's attractiveness.

More studies are needed to analyse the effect of programmes in relation to the characteristics of the participants (e.g. age, self-efficacy levels, etc.). Vocational education students represent a significant yet difficult-to-reach population. At present, surprisingly little attention has been given to this group who are at a high risk of becoming smokers (Corcoran and Allegrante, 1989). At present one European study has focussed on this group in particular and has found positive effects (de Vries, 1989). The programme providers vary from project staff or trained teachers to older or same-aged peer leaders. They need a thorough training and they should be non-smokers. Some settings in which the programme takes place, such as where there are high smoking levels and non-smoking school policies, may decrease the impact of prevention programmes. The effects are also dependent on the context in which a programme is delivered, such as the amount of health education provided in schools or communities.

Studies on the effects show a generally consistent pattern: after an experimental group has received the programme, smoking incidence is lower compared to a control group. Botvin (1986) concludes that the reported results generally range from reductions of 33% to 39% of the proportion of new smokers, 29% to 67% reduction of experimental smoking (less than one cigarette per week), and 43% to 47% reduction with regard to regular smoking (at least one cigarette per week). Small effects of smoking prevention programmes on quitting have been reported by some studies as well (Best et al., 1988).

The reported effects, however, become smaller at longer follow-ups. Two studies showed that the initial results did not last after six years (Flay et al., 1989; Murray et al., 1989). However, it is premature to conclude that only short-term effects can be achieved. A better conclusion is that smoking prevention research has been able to show modest short-term effects. Probably a variety of other activities are needed to maintain these results. Perhaps the answer is not to provide just booster sessions on non-smoking which may lead to boredom for non-smokers, but to embed smoking prevention in a broader health programme. Moreover, it may be unrealistic to expect enduring changes from a programme of a few lessons when adolescents are also confronted with so many pro-smoking messages in and outside schools.

Smoking prevention: other strategies

The issue of young people smoking must, therefore, be seen in a larger context of society's attitudes towards tobacco. Preventive efforts should be directed towards youngsters but also to the community as a whole. We will discuss other strategies to encourage non-smoking in youngsters below.

A spiral curriculum approach

Information on non-smoking should be embedded in a larger context, focusing on health, and should address other relevant health issues (UICC, 1990). As schools have limited time available, priorities have to be made by identifying health issues with common determinants (e.g. peer pressure) to increase economy of effort and likelihood of curricula adoption (Glynn, 1989).

Out-of-school activities

Reinforcing non-smoking within schools will not reach those who do not attend school any more, while it may be counter-productive for some who associate school with negative values. For these groups, it is essential to develop activities which are not associated with school.

Public information campaigns

Mass-media approaches can play a role in changing public attitudes about smoking. To be most effective they have to be developed in conjunction with educational and community-based programmes as well as legislation to change smoking behaviours.

Community approaches

These interventions aim to change behaviour by focusing on the community as a whole. Existing social networks of a community are used to develop and implement the programme. As a result, the community becomes involved, a feeling of 'ownership' with the programme will develop, and several sectors of the community will be included

(WHO, 1988; UICC, 1990). A non-smoking community programme can have special positive effects on youngsters. Firstly, it becomes more evident that a community norm will be in favour of non-smoking. Secondly, a broad social network may be essential for youngsters who encounter much social pressure to smoke from their environment. Therefore, anti-smoking activities for the social environment, such as cessation programmes for their parents, are needed as well. Finally, community programmes will probably have a greater chance of reaching the so-called drop-outs.

Smoking cessation programmes for adolescents

As smoking prevention programmes are not effective for all adolescents and do not reach all youngsters, we need to develop cessation programmes for adolescents. The factors determining quitting are highly similar to those described in Figure 2. Quitting is related with a more positive attitude towards non-smoking, with less social pressure towards smoking and with higher levels of self-efficacy towards non-smoking (de Vries, 1989). Moreover, stronger price policies and a better legislation may help young people quit (UICC, 1990).

Legislation and health policies

Several types of legislation should be introduced to promote non-smoking in youngsters (UICC, 1990):

(a) banning of all tobacco advertisements and promotion activities;

(b) reduction of the land committed to tobacco growth;

(c) smoke-free areas;

(d) legislation to increase tobacco prices. (In Hong Kong, tobacco prices quadrupled in 1983 and the number of teenage smokers halved between 1982 and 1984. In some Australian and US states, income from tax is used for health promotion funds);

(e) prominent and explicit disease warnings;

(f) banning of all new tobacco-related products. (Legislation to protect the public from unsafe products can be used to ban new tobacco-related products);

(g) prevention of selling cigarettes singly or in very small packets;

(h) mandatory health education for primary and secondary schools with the inclusion of smoking prevention.

European smoking prevention activities

Many European countries make attempts to prevent adolescents' smoking.

School-based smoking prevention

In most European countries, schools have been the setting for anti-smoking education. Many recently developed programmes include the three essential content components already described.

In 1984, in Northern England, a three-phase family-linked smoking prevention programme was developed (Charlton, 1986). The biology of smoking was presented to nine-year-old children, the social aspects and the problem of advertising were presented to 12-year-olds, and a 'stop-smoking' package developed for 15 and 16-year-olds. The programme for the nine-year-olds has been evaluated and the results show that fewer boys in the experimental group (5%) than in the control group (12%) have tried smoking since the pre-test.

A two-year intervention was developed in 1978 by the Finnish North Karelia Youth Project (Vartiainen *et al.*, 1986; 1990). The multi-component programme was delivered to 13-year-olds in the classroom by slightly older peer leaders. The results after two years showed that 27% and 26% of the students in the two intervention groups and 37% of the students in the reference area reported smoking at least monthly. Six years after the

programme the proportion of smokers in the two intervention groups was 38% and 31%, while in the reference group the proportion of smokers was 42%.

The Norwegian Oslo Youth Study (Tell *et al.*, 1984) used a similar approach to the former project. The intervention was delivered by the staff and student leaders. Apart from the usual topics, the content also covered coping with social anxiety, pressure-resistance training, self pollution and waste of resources, passive smoking, marketing of tobacco, and the fact that smoking is an individual choice. A two-year follow-up indicated that there were fewer new smokers among students who participated in the programme (16.5%) than in the control group (26.9%).

In the Netherlands, a smoking prevention programme for 13 and 14-year-olds was developed in 1985 (de Vries, 1989; de Vries and Dijkstra, 1989). The programme has five lessons and a video-peer-led design. After one year, 41.7% of high school attenders who had never smoked had experimented with smoking versus 52.1% in the control group. Effects on regular smoking among vocational students increased by 6.7% in the experimental group compared with 15.9% in the control group. Moreover, more treatment (17.9%) than control group (6.8%) smokers had reduced or quit smoking. The results of a two-year follow-up still favoured an impact on regular smoking in vocational students (de Vries *et al.*, 1990).

In Italy, a school-based smoking prevention programme developed for 15 to 17-year-olds did not seem to prevent the start of smoking (Figa-Talamanca and Modolo, 1989).

Smoking cessation programmes

At present two pilot studies on smoking cessation in the United Kingdom show promising results – a programme for 15 to 19-year-old smokers and a cessation programme for 15 and 16-year-olds in three high schools in Northern Ireland (the Belfast Project).

Activities outside the schools

Some European countries organize smoking prevention activities outside schools to enhance the attention of non-smokers to their non-smoking behaviour, such as a teenage magazine for young people in the UK and Ireland (WHO, 1988). Smokebuster clubs for nine to 13-year-olds which originate in the UK are now also starting up in Portugal, Ireland, Belgium and Australia (McTernan, 1990); similar activities are available in France ('Pataclope') and Scandinavia (the Smoke Free Generation group). However, studies on the effectiveness of these approaches are not yet available.

Legislation

Many countries in Europe have legislation prohibiting or restricting smoking in schools and other establishments used by young people, restrictions on sales of tobacco products to young people either through age (e.g. over 16 years) or through outlets (e.g. vending machines), or both. These restrictions are not always effective because they are often not fully implemented and are difficult to enforce. In some European countries, tobacco prices have been pushed up. In many countries, advertising and promotion is banned completely or partially, and disease warnings appear on tobacco packages and advertisements (WHO, 1989). Although the impact of legislative measures is hard to assess, it is agreed that it helps to promote smoking prevention and cessation (UICC, 1990).

Continuation of prevention

Several diffusion strategies can be developed for dissemination, adoption, implementation and maintenance of smoking prevention activities. For the dissemination of programmes, a good infra-structure is required. It is essential that the determinants of adoption, implementation and maintenance of a programme by the users and the target group are studied before the actual development of a programme in order to attune the programme to their wishes.

Rogers (1983) has listed several characteristics that will decrease the chances of adoption and implementation, such as complexity and high costs of the programme. With respect to adoption, three groups can be distinguished: the adopters, the majority and the laggards. Adopters can be reached easily by mass media information as they are more innovative minded. They can serve as a role model for the other groups (Bandura, 1989). The majority is more influenced by interpersonal information. The laggards are those who are reached with the greatest difficulty and who often need a very personal approach (Rogers, 1983).

To enhance diffusion, a linkage approach is advocated by Orlandi (1989) in which three groups can be distinguished. The resource group develops the materials for the target group that consists of both the users of the programme and the group who has to change their behaviour. The linkage group consists of representatives of both groups. The main function of this latter group is to develop and implement the intervention by taking into account relevant aspects and wishes of the resource and target group.

Apart from diffusion strategies, we also need supportive and health promotion policies facilitating actual and continued use of successful interventions. To enhance adoption and continued use, smoking prevention should be mandatory for secondary schools.

A broad health promotion and intersectoral approach will also enhance smoking prevention, as this enhances social support from several other organizations (e.g. the Ministry of Education).

Conclusions

Effective school-based smoking prevention programmes can be developed. However, most programmes have been developed as part of a research project and are not being widely used in schools. Consequently, the total impact of these programmes will be limited. We therefore need to focus more explicitly on the diffusion and adoption of well evaluated programmes by schools. Research should focus on the factors determining diffusion, adoption, and continued use of these programmes (see also Parcel *et al.*, 1989; Steckler *et al.*, 1989).

References

Ajzen, I. and Fishbein, M. (1980) *Understanding attitudes and predicting social behaviour*, Prentice Hall, Englewood Cliffs.

Bandura, A. (1986) *Social foundations of thought and action: a social cognitive theory*, Prentice Hall, New York.

Best, J.A., Thomson, S.J., Santi, S.M., Smith, E.A. and Brown, K.S (1988) Preventing cigarette smoking among school children, *Ann. Rev. Public Hlth.* **9**, 161–201.

Botvin, G.J (1986) Substance abuse prevention research: recent developments and future directions, *J. School Health* **9**, 369–374.

Corcoran, R.D. and Allegrante, J.P (1989) Vocational education students: a difficult-to-reach population at risk for smoking related cancer, *J. School Health* **59**, 195–198.

Charlton, A. (1986) Evaluation of a family-linked smoking programme in primary schools, *Health Ed. J.* **45**, 140–144.

De Vries, H. (1989a) *Smoking prevention in Dutch adolescents*, Datawyse, Maastricht.

De Vries, H. (1989b) *Who are the successful quitters?* Paper prepared for the International Union Against Cancer for the International Workshop on Children and Tobacco in Industrialized Countries, Toronto, Canada.

De Vries, H. and Dijkstra, M. (1989) Non-smoking: your choice, a Dutch smoking prevention programme – a case study. In James, C., Balding, J. and Harris, D. (eds.) *World yearbook of education 1989: health education*, Kogan Page, London, 20–31.

De Vries, H., Dijkstra and Kok, G.J. (1990) The effects of a Dutch peer-led smoking prevention programme on video. In Jamrozik, K. *Abstract book of the 7th World Conference on Tobacco and Smoking, 1–5 April, Perth, Australia*, 277.

Evans, R.I., Rozelle, R.M., Mittelmark, M.B., Hansen, W.B., Bane, A.L. and Havis, J. (1978) Deterring the onset of smoking in children: knowledge of immediate physiological effects and coping with peer pressure, media pressure and parent modeling, *J. App. Soc. Psychol.* **8**, 126–135.

Figa-Talamanca, I. and Modolo, M.A. (1989) Evaluation of an antismoking educational programme among adolescents in Italy, *HYGIE* **8**, 24–28.

Flay, B.R., Kopeke, D., Thomson, S.J., Santi, S., Best, J.A. and Brown, S. (1989) Six year follow-up of the first Waterloo school smoking prevention trial, *Am. J. Public Health* **79**, 1371–1376.

Glynn, T.J. (1989) Essential elements of school-based smoking prevention programmes, *J. School Health* **59**, 181–188.

Kok, G.J. and De Vries, H. (1989) Primary prevention of cancers: the need for health education and intersectoral health promotion. In Heller, T., Davey, B. and Bailey, L. (eds.), *Reducing the risk of cancers*, Hodder and Stoughton, Sevenoaks, 99-111.

Kok, G.J. and Green, L.W. (1990) Research to support health promotion in practice: a plea for increased cooperation, *Health Promotion International* **5**, 303–308.

McTernan, V. (1990) *Introduction to smokebusters*. Paper presented at the Conference on Young People and Tobacco, Glasgow, Scottish Committee Action on Smoking and Health, Edinburgh.

Leventhal, H. and Cleary, P.D. (1980) The smoking problem: a review of the research and theory in behavioural risk modification, *Psychological Bulletin* 88, 370–405.

Orlandi, M.A., Landers, C., Weston, R. and Haley, N. (1990) In Glanz, K., Lewis, F.M. and Rimer, B.K. (eds.) *Health behaviour and health education: theory, research and practice*, Jossey-Bass Publishers, San Francisco, 228–313.

Murray, D.M., Pirie, P., Luepker, R.V. and Pallonen, U. (1989) Five and six year follow-up results from four seventh-grade smoking prevention strategies, *J. Behavioural Med.* 12, 207–218.

Parcel, G.S., Eriksen, M.P., Lovato, C.Y., Gottlieb, N.H., Brink, S.G. and Green, L.W. (1989) The diffusion of school-based tobacco-use prevention programmes: project description and baseline data, *Health Ed. Res.* 4, 111–124.

Rogers, E.M. (1983) *Diffusion of innovations*, The Free Press, New York.

Steckler, A., McLeroy, K.R., Goodman, R.M., Smith, D., Dawson, L. and Howell, K. (1989) The importance of school district policies in the dissemination of tobacco use curricula in North Carolina Schools, *Family Community Hlth.* 12, 14–25.

Tell, G.S., Klepp, K.I., Vellar, O.D. and McAlister, A. (1984) Preventing the onset of cigarette smoking in Norwegian adolescents: The Oslo Youth Study, *Preventive Med.* 68, 256–275.

Thomson, E.L. (1978) Smoking education programmes 1960–1976, *Am. J. Public Health* 68, 250–257.

Tobler, N.S. (1986) Meta-analysis of 143 adolescents drug prevention programmes: quantitative outcome results of programme participants compared to a control or comparison group, *J. of Drug Issues* 16, 537–567.

UICC (1990) *A manual on tobacco and young people for the industrialised world*, International Union Against Cancer (UICC), Geneva.

Vartiainen, E., Pallonen, U., McAlister, A., Koskela, K. and Puska, P. (1986) Four-year follow-up results of the smoking prevention programme in the North Karelia Youth Project, *Preventive Med.* 15, 692–698.

Vartiainen, E., Pallonen, U., McAlister, A. and Puska, P. (1990) Eight-year follow-up results of an adolescent smoking prevention programme: The North Karelia Youth Project, *Am. J. Public Health* 80, 78–79.

WHO (1988) *Planning for a smoke-free generation, Smoke-Free Europe, Vol. 6*, WHO Regional Office for Europe, Copenhagen.

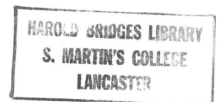
HAROLD BRIDGES LIBRARY
S. MARTIN'S COLLEGE
LANCASTER

BREAST SELF-EXAMINATION

Joan Austoker and Julie Evans

Breast cancer – an important health problem

Breast cancer is a disease that occurs mainly in western developed countries, with half the cases in the world occurring in North America and Europe (which contains less than one-fifth of the female world population) (Cancer Research Campaign, 1988). Throughout Europe, breast cancer is the most common cancer amongst women, comprising an estimated 25% of all cancer cases and 18% of all cancer deaths. Figure 1 shows that there is a wide range of incidence rates throughout the European Community, ranging from 39 per 100,000 women in Spain to 75 per 100,000 in the UK and Ireland (Moller Jensen *et al.*, 1990). Each year, over 15,000 women die from the disease in the UK and there are 25,000 new cases. The incidence of breast cancer rises from less than 10 per 100,000 women aged under 30 years to 300 per 100,000 in women aged over 85 years, and it is estimated that 1 in 12 women in the UK will develop breast cancer at some time in their life (Cancer Research Campaign, 1988).

The cause of breast cancer is not known. Therefore there is no immediate hope of prevention. Advances in treatments have achieved only modest improvements on survival, and on average two-thirds of women in the UK who develop the disease are likely to die from it. However, the stage at which a woman has her breast cancer diagnosed greatly influences her survival chances. In general, the earlier breast cancer is diagnosed, the better the chances of survival. The only remaining approach to solving the problem of breast cancer is therefore to achieve diagnosis at the earliest possible stage.

There are three potential methods of population screening for the early detection of breast cancer: mammography (or breast x-ray); clinical breast examination carried out by a doctor or nurse; and self-examination carried out by women themselves. In 1986, an examination of the evidence from a number of countries on the value of screening for breast cancer by all of these means was published in the UK (DHSS, 1986). The report concluded that only in the case of mammographic screening was there unequivocal evidence of a reduction in mortality. Breast cancer mortality could be reduced by up to one-third for women aged 50 and over who had undergone mammographic screening. On the basis of this report, the UK government launched in 1988 the first nationwide programme of mammographic screening for breast cancer for women aged 50 and over.

Whilst mammography is the preferred option for population screening for breast cancer, it is, however, not available to the majority of women in Europe nor to women aged under 50 in the UK. Clinical breast examination is not widely offered on a regular basis and therefore breast self-examination (or BSE) remains the best available means of early detection for most women.

What is BSE?

The recommended BSE techniques involve both inspection and systematic palpation of the breasts in a variety of postures. It is suggested that BSE should be conducted regularly once a month. For premenopausal women this should be at the same point in the menstrual cycle, preferably following the end of the menstrual period, because of the normal changes in breast tissue occurring during the cycle. Post-menopausal women should choose a convenient but consistent day in the month, for example the first.

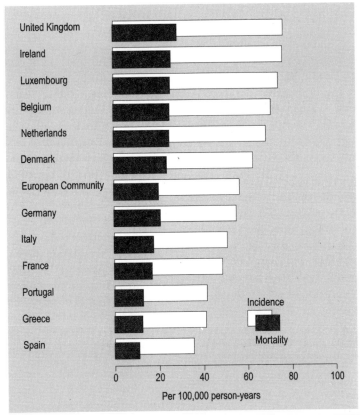

Figure 1 Estimated incidence and mortality of cancer of the female breast

Signs and symptoms that should be reported to a doctor without delay include: any changes in size or shape of a breast or nipple; any unusual lump or thickening of the skin; any dimpling or puckering of the skin or nipple; any nipple discharge or bleeding; any veins standing out more than usual.

The value of BSE

BSE has not in the past been subjected to the same critical appraisal as mammography, that is by means of a randomized controlled trial. A prospective randomized trial of BSE was launched in the USSR in 1983, where women had received no previous education about BSE (Semiglazov, 1987). A sample of women aged 40 to 64 years with no previous history of breast cancer was recruited to the study through health-care clinics in Leningrad and

Moscow. The clinics were randomly allocated to BSE education versus none. The teaching sessions consisted of a talk given by a trained nurse or doctor to groups of 5 to 20 women, and including a demonstration of breast examination on one of the women. Each woman was given a leaflet describing BSE technique, and a calendar to remind her to conduct BSE monthly.

After the first 15 months of the study in the Leningrad centres, more than twice as many breast cancers had been diagnosed in the BSE group as in the control group (1.15 per 1000 women compared with 0.51 per 1000 women), and the average size of the tumours detected was 1.3 cm smaller in the BSE group. However, an interim report in 1991 shows no difference in the number of cancers in the BSE and control groups (3.15 per 1000 women compared with 3.19 per 1000 women)

(Semiglazov, 1991). Moreover, BSE teaching sessions resulted in 'a higher frequency of visits to specialists with complaints about the "pathology" of the breast, a higher rate of reference to a specialized institution for an examination, and a higher number of the excision biopsies due to a benign lesion as compared with control'. The full results of this trial comparing mortality from breast cancer in the BSE and control groups will become available in 1994.

In the meantime, a series of studies have been reported in the literature which set out to relate the practice of BSE prior to development of breast cancer with stage of disease at diagnosis. Twelve of these studies were combined in a meta-analysis such that the statistical power and direction of results of each study contributed to a single overall estimate of effect (Hill *et al.*, 1988). When reported individually, six of the studies had shown some benefit of BSE and six had not.

Measures of BSE practice and extent of disease varied between studies. In some the extent of disease was related to patients' self-reported history of BSE practice before their illness, and in others women were questioned specifically whether their tumour had been found while doing BSE or accidentally. The combined results from six studies concerned with the patients' prior history of BSE suggest a beneficial effect of premorbid BSE practice on the degree of disease positive lymph nodes at diagnosis with a high degree of statistical significance. The effect is not so clear cut however for studies of the method of detection. This favourable result may be partly due to the effect of length bias, whereby benign tumours which may grow more slowly present a greater opportunity of detection when small or before nodes are affected (Day, 1988).

Only one of the 12 studies showed a statistically significant survival benefit amongst BSE performers (75% at five years versus 57% for non-performers) (Foster and Costanza, 1984). This survival benefit persisted in all age groups after controlling the analysis for confounding factors, such as family history of breast cancer, delay in treatment and method of detection. This beneficial effect can partly be explained by lead-time bias, whereby earlier detection produces a longer survival time from detection to death, whilst the course of the disease remains unaltered. Based on studies of breast tumour kinetics, the authors estimated a mean lead-time of approximately six months associated with BSE performance as opposed to a mean lead-time for mammographic screening of one to two years. Using estimates of lead-time in increments of six months the statistically significant survival benefit in BSE performers persisted even with lead-time estimates of up to three years. The authors concluded that the survival differences observed between BSE performers and non-performers could not therefore be explained solely on the basis of lead-time bias.

Further evidence for a beneficial effect of BSE was obtained from a prospective study of the effect of BSE on breast cancer mortality conducted in Nottingham (Locker *et al.*, 1989). Women in the study population were invited to attend educational sessions given by trained nurses and radiographers, consisting of a talk and film followed by discussion. Emphasis was placed on both visible and physical signs, the need for regular monthly examinations and the need to report immediately any changes noticed to specially set-up self-referral clinics. Mortality from breast cancer in the study group was compared with that in an historical control population from the same district prior to the introduction of BSE education. Survival data from breast cancer cases diagnosed in both groups showed no significant difference after seven years of follow-up.

However, analysis of the study population alone showed a significant survival advantage to those patients who attended the BSE education sessions prior to their tumour diagnosis compared to non-attenders. This beneficial effect of attendance for education was most marked in post-menopausal women. The study group contained more small (less than 2 cm), node negative and well differentiated tumours than the control group. Tumour size, grade and stage combined as a prognostic index demonstrated that 36% of study patients who developed breast cancer fell into a good prognostic group (i.e. having a better chance of cure) as against 27% of cases in the control group (Haybittle *et al.*, 1982).

Both this study and a similar study conducted in Huddersfield (Philip *et al.*, 1986) were undertaken as part of the UK Trial for the Early Detection of Breast Cancer (UKTEDBC) (DHSS, 1981). In the UKTEDBC breast cancer mortality was compared in two populations invited for annual mammographic screening, two populations invited to attend educational sessions about BSE, and four control populations offered no early detection services. The Huddersfield study, which was included in Hill's meta-analysis (Hill *et al.*, 1988), whilst showing a significant improvement in patient delay and clinical stage in BSE practitioners, did now show a significant difference in pathological status of axillary nodes between the study and control groups. The main results of the UKTEDBC reported in 1988 showed no significant difference in mortality between the BSE centres and the control centres (Chamberlain *et al.*, 1988).

A further study by Mant *et al.* (1987) confirmed earlier findings that premorbid BSE practice led to more favourable tumour characteristics at diagnosis. This beneficial effect of BSE was most marked in those women who had received formal instruction in BSE and practised it at least monthly. The effect of different types of training in BSE is not known; for example does provision of a leaflet lead to a different degree of improvement than instruction in a class or one-to-one sessions with a nurse or physician (O'Malley and Fletcher, 1987)?

Risks associated with BSE

The accuracy of BSE is dependent upon its sensitivity and specificity, sensitivity being the ability of the test to detect abnormalities in breast tissue, specificity being the ability to correctly detect cancerous abnormalities. O'Malley estimated the overall sensitivity of BSE using data from the Breast Cancer Detection Demonstration Project (BCDDP) to be 26% (O'Malley and Fletcher, 1987; Baker, 1982). This is poor compared to an estimated 75% for combined clinical breast examination and mammography. When broken down by age, BSE was found to be most sensitive for women aged 35 to 39 years (41%), and least sensitive for women aged 60 to 74 years (21%).

This is not surprising since breast lumps are more common in younger women, whose breasts are subject to the fluctuating hormone levels of the menstrual cycle (Devitt, 1977). Very few of these lumps, however, turn out to be malignant. In post-menopausal women, the likelihood of a lump being malignant is higher. A study by Devitt showed that 48% of lumps detected in a group of women aged over 55 were malignant, compared with 3% in women aged under 44 (Devitt, 1983). Therefore, younger women practising BSE may be subject to a less favourable balance of potential risks versus benefits.

It has been argued that women who find asymptomatic benign breast lesions by BSE are exposed to unnecessary anxiety, unnecessary medical investigations and potential risks of false reassurance (Frank and Mai, 1985). All breast symptoms require detailed investigation (including mammography and/or invasive procedures) to determine whether the lesions are benign or malignant. Thus women who do not have breast cancer will undergo such investigations and the associated inconvenience, discomfort and anxiety without experiencing any benefits. These investigative procedures are costly to provide. There is also a risk that women who have experienced one or more benign diagnoses may delay presentation of a further (possibly malignant) lump on the basis of their past experience (Frank and Mai, 1985).

Regular practice of BSE in itself can cause considerable anxiety in some women, because of the possibility that they will eventually find something suspicious. This may be one of many reasons why few women conduct regular BSE despite high levels of awareness of BSE in the population (O'Malley and Fletcher, 1987). In general the frequency of BSE performance is highest in younger, better educated women with higher incomes. Anxiety may also prevent women who have found 'something' from presenting their symptoms immediately, thereby reducing any possible benefit of early detection.

Another possible reason why some women are reluctant to practise BSE may be because they perceive BSE technique to be complicated, and have little confidence in their ability to do it correctly. To further the state of uncertainty about the benefits of BSE, there is no consensus on what constitutes a competent self-examination, or how frequently it should be carried out. There is a school of thought which believes that BSE could be made more acceptable to women if the concept of BSE were changed from that of a regular, ritualistic exercise following a set technique, to one in which breast examination was built into women's daily life experience. Women could be encouraged to take frequent and convenient opportunities to observe and feel their breasts, such as while washing or dressing, so as to become familiar with the texture of their normal breast tissue and how it changes during the menstrual cycle. They should become aware of any changes from this normal state, and report these promptly to their family doctor. This concept has become known as 'breast awareness'.

Conclusions

The promotion of BSE as a primary screening procedure is of unproven benefit (Mant, 1989). In consequence, the UK Department of Health Breast Screening Advisory Committee has recommended that BSE should not be regarded as a primary screening technique, but should be regarded as no more than an intervention which may have a beneficial but limited effect (Department of Health, 1989).

Because of the relatively high incidence of breast cancer in older women and the increased specificity of BSE in these women, it has been suggested by some that women attending mammographic screening programmes should be encouraged to practise BSE between mammographic screens (Foster and Costanza, 1984). Mammography is not a perfect or preventive procedure, and women should be made aware that breast cancer can develop at any time including during the period between screens. The situation with respect to younger women remains less clear.

The 'message' about BSE is still confused and ambiguous, and the variety and diversity of materials and practices across Europe remains considerable.

As Baines has stressed, crucial questions remain unanswered about BSE and will not be answered in a satisfactory manner in the absence of good randomized studies (Baines, 1988).

These questions are:

- By whom, where and how can very large numbers of women best be taught BSE?
- At what age is instruction in BSE appropriate?
- What are the minimum components essential for instilling effective practice of breast awareness?
- How frequently should BSE be performed?
- Is it feasible and practical to offer a programme of instruction?

- If a programme of instruction is instituted, what is the best way of reinforcing it?
- How can BSE performance be evaluated?
- How can the benefits and costs of BSE practice be measured?

In the absence of answers to these questions, research is currently being conducted in the UK under the auspices of the National Breast Screening Programme to review all the existing evidence and materials on BSE/breast awareness with a view to developing a clear and consistent UK policy for advising women of all ages.

References

Baines, C.J. (1988) Breast self examination: the known and the unknown. In Day, N.E. and Miller, A.B. *Screening for breast cancer*, Toronto, UICC, 85–91.

Baker, L.H. (1982) Breast cancer detection demonstration project. Five year summary report, *Cancer Ann.* **32**, 194–225.

Cancer Research Campaign (1988) *Breast cancer*, Cancer Research Campaign.

Chamberlain, J., Coleman, D., Ellman, R., Moss, S. *et al.*, (1988) First results on mortality reduction in the UK trial of early detection of breast cancer, *Lancet* **ii**, 411–416.

Day, N.E. (1988) Self examination of the breast (letter), *Brit. Med. J.* **297**, 624.

Department of Health Advisory Committee on Breast Screening (1989) Policy on BSE and breast awareness. In *Health education draft guidelines*, Screening Publications, Oxford.

Department of Health and Social Security (1986) *Breast Cancer Screening* (Forrest Report), HMSO, London.

Department of Health and Social Security Working Group (1981) UK trial of early detection of breast cancer: description of method, *Brit. J. Cancer*, **44**, 618–627.

Devitt, J. (1977) Value of this history in the office diagnosis of breast cancer, *Cancer Med. Assoc. J.* **116**, 1127–1128.

Devitt, J. (1983) How breast cancer presents, *Cancer Med. Assoc. J.* **129**, 43–7.

Foster, R.S.and Costanza, M.C. (1984) Breast self examination practices and breast cancer survival, *Cancer* **53**, 999–1005.

Frank, J. and Mai, V. (1985) BSE in young women: more harm than good? *Lancet* Sept 21, 654–657.

Haybittle, J.L., Blamey, R.W., Elston, C.W. *et al.* (1982) A prognostic index in primary breast cancer, *Brit. J. Cancer* **45**, 361.

Hill, D., White, V., Jolley, D.and Mapperson, K. (1988) Self examination of the breast: is it beneficial? Meta-analysis of studies investigating BSE and extent of disease in patients with breast cancer, *Brit. Med. J.* **297**, 271–275.

Locker, A.P., Caseldine, J., Mitchell, A.K., Blamey, R.W., Roebuck, E.J.and Elston, C.W. (1989) Results from a seven-year programme of BSE in 89010 women, *Brit. J. Cancer* **60**, 401–405.

Mant, D. (1989) Breast self examination. Should we discourage it? *J. Roy. Coll. Gen. Pract.* 180–181.

Mant, D., Vessey, M.P., Neil, A., McPherson, K.and Jones, L. (1987) BSE and breast cancer stage at diagnosis, *Brit. J. Cancer* **55**, 207–211.

Moller Jensen, O., Esteve, J., Moller, H. and Renard, H. (1990) Cancer in the European Community and its member states, *Euro. J. Cancer* **26** (no. 11/12), 1167–1256.

O'Malley, M.and Fletcher, S. (1987) Screening for breast cancer with BSE: a critical review, *J. Am. Med. Assoc.* 257, **(16)**, 2197–2203.

Philip, J., Harris, G., Flaherty, C. and Joslin, C.A.F. (1986) Clinical measures to assess the practice and efficiency of BSE, *Cancer* **58**, 973–977.

Semiglazov, V.F. (1991) *Role of BSE in early breast cancer: 5 year results of the USSR/WHO randomized study in Leningrad*. Abstract presented to the First EUSOMA International Conference, March 1991.

Semiglazov, V.F. and Moiseenko, V.M. (1987) BSE for the early detection of breast cancer: a USSR/WHO controlled trial in Leningrad, *Bulletin of the WHO* **65** (3), 391–396.

PART 4
INTEGRATED ACTION TO PREVENT CANCERS

Introduction

In many of the papers in this book it has been argued that action to prevent cancers and reduce the risk of individuals developing them is a multi-faceted activity which must take place at many different levels. It makes it easier for individuals to change if they live in societies and communities where multi-sectoral integrated activities for health promotion are taking place which make healthy choices easier. Social norms and expectations are prominent influences on people's behaviour. It is unlikely that someone trying to manage their health behaviour in the direction of lower risk will be able to do this without being influenced by the wider factors that are likely to help or hinder them in doing so.

In his paper 'Programme principles associated with successful health education and health promotion interventions', Donald Iverson outlines twenty basic principles of effective practice in health promotion drawn from the experience of health education programmes throughout the world. This provides a good base from which to consider effective integrated health promotion interventions.

The area where integrated multi-sectoral activity has been most comprehensively developed is that of anti-tobacco activity. In 'Co-ordinated action against tobacco', Patti White describes the ways in which this has been conducted. A major part of this activity has been directed not only at changing broad social attitudes towards tobacco, but also at bringing about legislative changes. Governmental action at national and international level is important in achieving a comprehensive tobacco policy whereby the dangers of products are publicized, tar yields are reduced, prices are increased by taxation,

and advertising is controlled. White highlights the importance of co-ordinated action across the European Community. It has taken a long time to bring this about and there is still much to do. Nonetheless, she shows evidence that it is possible to achieve major changes if there is the social and political will to do so. Many lessons can be learned from the campaign against tobacco for other areas of cancer prevention activities concerned, for example, with reducing alcohol consumption or improving the popular diet.

It is with diet and wider policies and practices impinging upon it that Verner Wheelock concerns himself in 'Food policy and cancers'. There are tensions and complex relationships between individual preferences, social dietary habits, income, price, economic vested interests, food producers, government policies and other factors. Mass retailers such as supermarkets and governments can both exert an influence on what is available for consumption by the general population. It is important to consider their role, as well as that of consumer pressure in trying to work towards a society in which healthy eating choices, along the lines suggested by the European Code Against Cancer, are more widely available to all sections of the community.

It is not necessary to wait until all answers are known and all methodological problems are solved before starting to act to prevent cancers. In 'Searching for consensus: a case study of rectal and colonic cancers', Allyson Pollock discusses one way in which provisional agreement can be reached over medical and scientific knowledge in cancer prevention. The consensus process aims to reach interim agreement about the knowledge and practice in particular areas so that patients can be treated in the most effective way before definitive answers are reached to complex problems. Even in a circumscribed field such as the prevention of colonic and rectal cancers it is not easy to ensure that a representative consensus is reached. Ordinary people who are the recipients of practice determined by a consensus process may find it difficult to have an effective voice in this process, while the powerful voice of the medical profession often continues to dominate the proceedings.

PROGRAMME PRINCIPLES ASSOCIATED WITH SUCCESSFUL HEALTH EDUCATION AND HEALTH PROMOTION INTERVENTIONS

Donald C. Iverson

Introduction

We have formulated 20 programme principles which we believe characterize many of the successful efforts to modify behaviour. If the suggested principles are considered when designing health education programmes, the likelihood of the programmes achieving their desired behaviour changes should be increased. Formulation of these programme principles does not imply that additional research on issues directly related to the principles is not necessary; rather, it implies that if further research on these principles is conducted, the studies should be designed to increase our understanding of how the principles apply in different settings and with different populations.

Principle 1: Health education programmes directed at large populations yield significant public health effects.

The question is often raised whether health education programmes should be directed at the general population or only at those persons considered to be at high risk for the problem. A combination of the population and high-risk strategies should be used, as these strategies have independent and additive effects (Lewis *et al.*, 1986). Also, rather than attempting to eliminate a single risk behaviour, a more effective approach is to achieve modest reductions in multiple risk behaviours within the total population (Kottke *et al.*, 1985).

While the overall percent reduction is often small when a population approach is used, the number of persons affected is large. For example, in the North Karelia pilot programme 0.5% of smokers quit and

remained abstinent at six months, and between 1% and 2% of persons reported losing weight. This amounted to 5,000 and 60,000 persons, respectively (Puska *et al.*, 1981). A smoking cessation programme in Canada utilizing television and community organization produced a 2.9% reduction in smoking, or 8,800 fewer smokers than expected (Millar and Naegele, 1987). The 'Quit For Life' programme in Sydney, Australia, produced only a 2.8% reduction in smoking prevalence that translated into 83,000 fewer smokers (Dwyer *et al.*, 1986; Pierce *et al.*, 1986). In the United States, the rather diffuse anti-smoking campaign that occurred between the years 1964 to 1978 resulted in the avoidance of over 200,000 premature smoking-related deaths, with many more deaths expected to be avoided in the 1980s and 1990s as either a direct or indirect result of the campaign (Warner and Murt, 1983).

Principle 2: The most efficacious health education programmes are often the least cost-effective.

Health education programmes are often researched in highly controlled situations in order to ensure that any changes are due to the programme itself and not some other factor. Additionally, many resources are used in the design and implementation of the programmes in order to maximize the likelihood of achieving the desired behaviour goals. These programmes generally produce the greatest effects, but at a considerable resource cost. Because of the resources required, these programmes usually have to be modified prior to their use on a wide-scale basis. Since most of the programmes as originally developed utilize multiple health education strategies, it is unclear which of the strategies can be eliminated or modified without risking a significant reduction in the programme's effects. The challenge is to identify health education programmes that produce an acceptable level of change at an acceptable cost (i.e. cost-effective) minimal intervention.

For example, combining a self-help manual with a provider intervention produced two to three times more non-smokers at six months than did the provider intervention alone (Janz et al., 1987). A minimal intervention weight-loss programme produced results equal to a more lengthy behavioural intervention (Black et al., 1984) and a worksite weight-loss programme that was directed by volunteers was as effective as a programme directed by professional leaders (Peterson et al., 1985).

In the first example, the combined approach is probably the most cost-effective because of the increased impact and the low cost of the additional intervention. In the latter two examples, the minimal interventions were the most cost-effective since they produced results statistically similar to the more intensive interventions. While these examples are encouraging, they may be the exception rather than the norm. For example, it is unlikely that the impressive results of the STARR programme in Kansas City should be matched or even approximated with a 'minimal' version of the programme (Pentz, Dwyer et al., 1989).

There are, however, instances when programmes which produce the lowest overall effects are the most cost-effective. A self-help approach for smoking cessation produced lower quitting rates than a smoking cessation class or an incentive-based quit smoking contest, but was still the most cost-effective of the three approaches (Altman et al., 1987). Worksite weight loss competitions result in lower long-term success rates than more intensive weight loss programmes, but are nonetheless the most cost-effective (Stunkard et al., 1989). However, if the impact of a

minimal intervention is quite small compared to a more intensive intervention, it will probably not be the most cost-effective approach (Davis et al., 1984).

Principle 3: The reasons underlying individual decisions to initiate behaviour change are varied. Many are not directly related to health.

There is little evidence that health is a salient value for most individuals. Rather, it seems that the importance of health rises for an individual when health conditions occur that interfere with important aspects of the individual's life (e.g. a hearing condition interferes with an individual's ability to listen to music). In addition, a number of disparate factors appear to be predictive of health behaviour (Cleary, 1984). Thus, health education programmes must address both health and non-health issues if they hope to attract and impact the members of a target population. This is precisely the approach used in most of the school-based smoking prevention and cessation programmes.

A number of examples can be used to illustrate the concept of multiple motivations. For example, an examination of the combined effects of economics and the presence of symptoms or clinical signs on women having a mammogram found that both had a significant effect, with economics having a greater impact when there were no symptoms or clinical signs present (Lane, 1983).

Employees participating in a worksite fitness programme cited a number of reasons for starting and remaining in the programme, including health-related, appearance-related, social-related, and emotional-related reasons (Iverson et al., 1989). The level of satisfaction with one's health and one's stated desire to make behaviour changes did not predict participation in worksite health promotion programmes (Davis et al., 1987); and an individual's selection of which health behaviours to change when a change was desired was often not related to the actual importance of that behaviour to personal health status (Levenkron and Greenland, 1988).

Principle 4: Personalizing health information affects the motivation/commitment phase of behaviour change.

It has long been assumed that people react more favourably to health information when it relates to their personal health status. For example, the majority of physician-based smoking interventions now include a step in which the physician delivers a message relating the patient's smoking to his or her health status (Glynn and Manley, 1989). Health risk appraisal instruments represent one of the most comprehensive approaches for providing individuals with detailed information about the effects of their lifestyle on various health status measures.

While health risk appraisal instruments have a modest direct impact on behaviour (Beery *et al.*, 1981), they do appear to affect the cognitive and affective determinants of behaviour change (Godin *et al.*, 1987). Thus, it appears that personalizing health information increases the likelihood of behaviour change by affecting the motivation/commitment phase (Marlatt and Gordon, 1985), or other pre-contemplation or contemplation stages of behaviour change. In some instances, personalized health information may be the cue that results in a behaviour change attempt, or it may function as a reinforcer of a recent behaviour change.

Principle 5: Programme participants possess characteristics that differ from those of non-participants.

Individuals who choose to participate in a health programme, regardless of the programme's structure, are different in important ways from individuals who elect not to participate in the programme. For example, programme participants may have lifestyles that are healthier than those of non-participants (Atkins *et al.*, 1987), or

participants and non-participants may have similar lifestyle habits but differ with respect to other characteristics, such as age and perceptions about personal health (Zavela *et al.*, 1988).

The type and focus of the programme also affects who will participate. In a community-based coronary heart disease prevention programme, women preferred group classes while men preferred self-help approaches. Exercise and smoking cessation classes were more popular among individuals under 40 years of age while weight loss and nutrition programmes were more popular among persons of 40 to 59 years of age (Lefebvre, Harden *et al.*, 1987). Similar findings have been reported for adolescents (Ferguson *et al.*, 1989).

It appears that a few variables may explain a majority of the variance between participants and non-participants (Pirie *et al.*, 1986). If these variables can be identified shortly after a programme has been offered to the target population, it should be possible to make adjustments to the programme in order to attract persons who otherwise would not participate.

Principle 6: Principles of diffusion theory apply to programme acceptance and programme participation rates.

Diffusion theory suggests that individuals can be placed into categories depending on when they are likely to adopt an innovation. The rate of adoption can be increased by using a combination of mass media and interpersonal channels to disseminate information about the innovation to individuals in the various adopter categories, and by modifying select aspects of the innovation itself (Rogers and Shoemaker, 1971).

Principles of diffusion theory have been considered in the design and implementation of many health education programmes. In the North Karelia programme, communication strategies were selected based on their ability to affect steps of the adoption process (Puska *et al.*, 1985). The importance of using different communication strategies had been previously demonstrated in the Stanford Three-Community study (Farquhar, 1978).

In the Pawtucket project, special attention was paid to the characteristics of an innovation that would affect its rise of adoption (Lefebvre, Lasater *et al.*, 1987). Yet, while systematically addressing select principles of diffusion theory in community-based health projects increases the likelihood of programme success (McLeroy *et al.*, 1988; Monahan and Scheirer, 1988, Murray, 1986), far too often health programmes are planned and implemented without serious consideration to diffusion theory.

Principle 7: Mass media have a modest effect on behaviour change; however, mass media do affect the initial phases of the behaviour change process.

Mass media have important roles to play in any health education programme directed at individuals, groups or communities. Among their primary roles are increasing awareness, generating interest, providing specific information, and setting the health agenda. While mass media are known to affect the initial phases of the behaviour change process, they can also result in actual behaviour change. The degree of success mass media can have in eliciting behaviour changes is dependent upon their duration and intensity, as well upon the target population's level of readiness for change. In many instances, mass media produce benefits long after the formal programme has been completed (Warner and Murt, 1983).

Mass media alone produce modest levels of behaviour change. For example, media-based smoking control programmes have been known to increase non-smoking prevalence by an average of 8% (Flay, 1987) as well as encouraging a significant number of people to reduce the number of cigarettes they smoke (Millar and Naegele, 1987; Pierce *et al.*, 1986). However, as previously stated, modest successes can translate to a large impact if the programme is directed at the general population.

Principle 8: For mass media to be effective, they must be intensive and prolonged; when mass media are combined with community programmes their effectiveness is increased.

At any one time, individuals are at varying places along the behaviour change continuum (Marlatt and Gordon, 1985; Prochaska, 1989). As a result, mass media will differentially affect individuals in the target population. Some individuals will take a long time to respond. Thus for mass media-based messages to affect a significant portion of the population, they must be sustained for a period sufficient to ensure that a majority of the population will be exposed to the message on a number of occasions.

When a mass media programme is part of a more comprehensive programme, its impact on behaviour change rates is increased. This was initially demonstrated in the Stanford Three-Community Study (Farquhar *et al.*, 1977). When mass media are combined with other community programmes, there is a two-to three-fold increase in effect (Flay, 1987). Mass media also appear to increase the effectiveness of school-based health education programmes (Flay, 1986; Pentz, Brannon *et al.*, 1989). It is possible that the addition of multiple community programmes to complement mass media may further increase the overall effectiveness of the programme. For example, when a self-help group was added to a mass media campaign which was already supplemented by self-help materials, there was a doubling of the programme's effects (Jason *et al.*, 1987).

Principle 9: Most community programmes are based on a number of theoretical constructs; it is not possible to identify which of the theoretical constructs is most important.

Community health promotion programmes are typically based on a variety of theories in such areas as community organization, behaviour change, or information processing, among others. In some programmes two or three theories dominate. In others, five or more theories are used. A further complication is that most programmes focus on select components of a theory; seldom, if ever, is a programme developed on the basis of all the components of a theory (Elder *et al.*, 1985; Lefebvre, Lasater *et al.*, 1987; Pentz, Dwyer *et al.*, 1989; Puska *et al.*, 1985). Thus, while community programmes have been shown to be effective in eliciting desired changes in behaviour, the independent contribution of each programme component or theoretical construct remains unknown.

Designing a community study to identify the independent contribution of each component or construct is probably not possible, and even if such a study could be done, the study's results would probably be of little value. Suggestions regarding which programme components or theoretical constructs are most important can be derived from multivariate and other analytic techniques, but only if reasonably accurate estimates of programme exposure are available. Similar problems are often encountered when behaviour change programmes are designed for individuals.

Principle 10: School health education programmes based on skills training, peer involvement, select components of social learning theory and involvement of the community produce the greatest changes.

A variety of health education approaches have been shown to be effective in eliciting behaviour changes among school-aged children and youth. Health education programmes designed to increase the student's basic life skills and personal competences in coping with social influences (Botvin and Eng, 1982), peer-led programmes focusing on social influences (Murray *et al.*, 1987), programmes based on development of interpersonal skills (Schinke *et al.*, 1985), and programmes based on social pressure

resistance skills (Johnson *et al.*, 1986) have all been shown to be effective.

Virtually all of the most effective programmes focus on skill acquisition, but the skills selected as the focus of the programmes often differ. For example, a programme could focus primarily on social pressure resistance skills (Johnson *et al.*, 1986), stress-management skills, decision-making skills or goal-setting skills. Other programme activities are often intended to increase levels of self-esteem (Hansen *et al.*, 1988). It is likely that different skills are needed to affect a health-enhancing behaviour, such as regular exercise vs. a health-deteriorating behaviour such as cigarette smoking, but it is also likely that there are a number of general skills that affect both types of behaviours.

Currently, a great deal is known about the approaches that are effective for smoking prevention programmes. Among the approaches shown to have an independent effect on smoking are peer pressure resistance training, correction of normative expectations, innoculation against mass media influences, information about parental and other adult influences, and peer leadership (Hansen *et al.*, 1988).

Principle 11: Combinations of educational/behavioural interventions delivered by physicians are more effective than individual interventions.

Principle 12: Physician-based programmes are most effective when the patient is exposed to the programme on a number of occasions.

In general, the greater the number of different interventions a patient receives from a physician and the more frequently a patient is exposed to any one physician-delivered intervention, the greater the impact of the intervention on the patient's behaviour (Kottke *et al.*, 1987; Ockene, 1987). However, there is no consistency in the magnitude of the effect when multiple interventions are used –

the effect can be less than additive, or synergistic. For example, adding nicotine gum to a short-term follow-up intervention increased smoking cessation from 3% to 22%, while adding nicotine gum to a long-term follow-up intervention increased cessation from 22% to 27% (Fagerstrom, 1984). The addition of a clinic support component to a brief smoking cessation intervention delivered by a physician increased the effect from 2.1% to 5.5% (Russell *et al.*, 1988). The differences in the magnitude of effect may be due to the dissimilarity of approaches among the combined interventions, patient preferences for the combined approaches, or the patient's readiness to change the target behaviour.

Recently, attempts have been made to synthesize the expanding literature on this topic by using meta-analytic techniques. Results of one meta-analysis indicate that adding counselling, self-help booklets and nicotine gum to physician advice results in significant reductions in patient smoking behaviour (Ockene, 1987). Another meta-analysis suggests that the level of success is dependent on the type of patient session (individual or group), the number of different interventions used, the number of sessions in which the target behaviour is reinforced and the number of months following the change in which the new behaviour is reinforced (Kottke *et al.*, 1987).

Principle 13: Self-help materials have a modest effect on behaviour; however, their effect is increased when they are combined with other interventions.

The magnitude of the expected effect on behaviour from self-help materials is somewhat dissimilar to the effect of mass media. If the materials give the person specific advice and help him or her acquire appropriate skills and if the person is predisposed to change or has recently made a behaviour change attempt, the materials will have a greater impact than if one or both of these conditions are absent. In smoking cessation, self-help materials have been shown

to be significantly more effective than placing people on a waiting list (Pederson *et al.*, 1981).

When self-help materials are reviewed with a patient by a therapist, the effect is similar to when the materials are merely given to the patient (Glasgow *et al.*, 1981). A self-help book on reducing drinking resulted in a greater reduction in the number of drinks consumed per week than did general advice and information about drinking (Heather *et al.*, 1987), but the addition of self-help materials to nicotine gum intervention did not result in an increase in smoking cessation rates (Lando *et al.*, 1988). In general, self-help materials appear to produce an independent and significant impact on behaviour. When well developed materials are used with appropriate individuals, the effect can be much higher than expected.

Principle 14: Individuals tend to change behaviours rapidly rather than slowly over time.

While most individuals take a long time becoming aware of the need for a behaviour change and an almost equally long period preparing for the change, once a decision has been made to change the behaviour, the rate of change is usually rapid rather than slow. For example, the vast majority of people attempting to stop smoking continue to use a 'cold turkey' approach. Individuals wanting to lose weight usually make significant changes in their diets in order to lose weight quickly, and people who decide to start an exercise programme often initiate exercise at too intense a level, resulting in significant muscle fatigue and soreness.

In the Women's Health Trial, participants were encouraged and taught to alter their diet systematically and slowly in order to reduce their percent of daily calories from fat from an average of 39% to an average of 20% over a 12-week period. In spite of the structured format of the intervention, most participants achieved a 20% calories as fat diet within two weeks (Insull *et al.*). Given this pattern of behaviour change, it may be necessary to help individuals develop behaviour change and maintenance skills early in the intervention.

Principle 15: Self-monitoring appears to enhance an individual's ability to initiate and sustain behaviour change.

Among the important functions of self-monitoring are collecting data necessary for the identification of the problem and opportunities for change, and reinforcing the person once the change(s) have been made. Self-monitoring is often an integral part of behavioural interventions and is increasingly used to reinforce behaviour changes. Self-monitoring has been shown to increase the number of lifestyle behaviours routinely practised (Bertera and Cuthie, 1984). Frequent self-monitoring (e.g. daily) is more effective than infrequent self-monitoring (e.g. less than weekly) (Bertera and Cuthie, 1984; King *et al.*, 1988). There is some evidence that the effects of self-monitoring can be generalized to different situations and to other behaviours (Koegel *et al.*, 1986). There are few instances in which individuals would not benefit from self-monitoring activities.

Principle 16: Environmental variables such as the number of alcohol outlets per capita influence the prevalence and the public health consequences of a behaviour.

Environmental variables can function as cues to behaviour change, facilitators of behaviour change, or reinforcers of behaviour change. Environmental variables can take many forms, including laws, regulations, community support and environmental modifications, such as cafeteria modification and construction of bicycle paths. While the literature supports the importance of environmental variables, the effect of these variables on health behaviour varies widely.

Increasing the drinking age from 18 to 21 years has been shown to reduce the number of alcohol-related deaths by 33% for persons aged 15 to 18 years and 38% for persons aged 19 and 20 years (Decker *et al.*, 1988). The number of retail and on-premise sites where alcohol can be purchased is correlated with cirrhosis mortality rates (Colon, 1981). If states were to restrict alcohol availability per capita, it has been estimated that consumption could be reduced by as much as two drinks per person per day (Hoadley *et al.*, 1984). Worksite smoking policies can reduce smoking prevalence and the number of cigarettes smoked (Peterson *et al.*, 1988). And if schools have a smoking policy that includes enforcement, a significant reduction in smoking behaviour is possible if the school also has prevention and cessation programme components (Pentz, Brannon *et al.*, 1989).

Legislation has had a significant effect on the use of seat belts and child restraints. In Germany, there was an increase in seat-belt use after the introduction of a law and a further increase in usage after a fine was added (Marburger and Friedel, 1987). In the United States, legislation has had an impact on the use of child restraints, but the effect across states ranges from significant increases to reductions in usage (Seekins *et al.*, 1988). The range of effect seems to be largely due to the level of enforcement and the consequences of conviction.

Modification of the environment has also been shown to influence behaviour. Posters in a cafeteria suggesting the benefits of a low-fat diet resulted in an increase in the purchase of low-fat entrées (Mayer *et al.*, 1986); prompts in a fast food restaurant increased the sales of salads (Wagner and Winett, 1988); and cafeteria point-of-purchase labelling resulted in a decrease in the purchase of foods high in calories, sodium and fat (Schmitz and Fielding, 1986). Other studies have shown few changes in dietary behaviour as a result of environmental interventions (Ernst *et al.*, 1986).

Principle 17: Behaviour relapse occurs rapidly, but individuals remain at risk for relapse for many years.

The process of sustained behaviour change usually involves a series of lapses and often, relapses (Marlatt and Gordon, 1985). When relapse occurs, it tends to occur within three months of the behaviour change attempt (Hunt and Bespalec, 1974). For example, in one study, 66% of smokers completing a cessation programme relapsed within three months; 40% of these persons relapsed in the week following cessation (Cummings et al., 1985). Since relapse can occur several months or even years after the initial behaviour change attempt (Glasgow and Lichtenstein, 1987; Pierce 1989), intensive follow-up efforts are necessary immediately following the behaviour change with some level of follow-up being required for a period of one or more years.

Principle 18: Relapse prevention components appear to be necessary to sustain behaviour change; however, little is known about the factors that influence relapse for specific behaviours.

While the importance of relapse prevention and behaviour maintenance efforts have been recognized by most researchers, little is known about which factors should be emphasized in an intervention. Among the factors affecting relapse from a weight loss regimen are a precipitating environmental or social event, a negative psychological state, a cycle of guilt and disparagement and a collapse of self-management behaviours (Brownell and Jeffery, 1987). Predictors of long-term abstinence for persons dependent on alcohol and heroin include social stability (especially employment), compulsory supervision, adoption of a substitute dependency, development of new relationships and association with an inspirational group (Vaillant, 1988).

Maintenance of positive health behaviours is associated with psychological well-being, subjective health status and a conventional behaviour orientation (Mechanic and Cleary, 1980). Translation of this knowledge into effective interventions remains a challenging task. For example, relapse prevention strategies based on social support have been shown to be effective but strategies based on the Marlatt and Gordon relapse prevention model have produced conflicting results (Curry et al., 1988; Glasgow and Lichenstein, 1987). Disappointing results have also occurred with weight-loss maintenance programmes (Perri et al., 1987). It is probable that greater understanding of how to design relapse prevention programmes will occur in the next few years as more research is now focussing on the issue.

Principle 19: Social support affects all phases of the behaviour change process.

Social support plays an important role in encouraging, facilitating and reinforcing behaviour change, and has even been shown to be a predictor of mortality (Berkman and Syme, 1979). As with most interventions, the magnitude of the effect of social support interventions ranges from little or no effect to a significant and substantial effect. For example, a social support component added to a cognitive-behaviour smoking-cessation intervention produced results in the anticipated direction, but the changes were not significant. On the other hand, a family-based social support intervention for hypertensives resulted in significant increases in appointment-keeping, weight control and blood-pressure control (Morisky et al., 1985).

The most successful social support interventions are likely to be those that match the type of social support (i.e. emotional support, appraisal support, informational support, instrumental support) to the various phases of the behaviour change process (Israel, 1985). For example, in a study on health care utilization patterns, low functional social supports were found to be associated with increased office visits, longer office visits, and higher annual health-care charges, while structural measures of social support were not related to any utilization indicator (Broadhead et al., 1989).

Principle 20: Participant characteristics appear to influence selection of, and success with, different interventions.

When interventions are matched to the needs and characteristics of participants, the likelihood of behaviour change increases. For example, nicotine gum tends to be more effective for persons who are highly nicotine dependent (Jarvik and Schneider, 1984). An externally focussed smoking-cessation intervention produced significantly greater results with externally focussed vs. internally focussed participants (Harackiewicz et al., 1987), and an alcohol-misuse prevention curriculum for elementary school students was effective only for students with prior supervised or unsupervised alcohol use (Dielman et al., 1989). Different factors have been shown to be predictive of participation, attrition and outcome for worksite smoking-cessation programmes (Klesges et al., 1988). Thus, pursuit of the ideal match between participant and programme characteristics, referred to as treatment/aptitude interaction, is likely to emerge as a major focus for research (Holloway et al., 1988).

References

Altman, D.G., Flora, J.A., Fortmann, S.P., and Farquhar, J.W. (1987) The cost-effectiveness of three smoking cessation programmes, *Am. J. Public Hlth.* **77**, 162–165.

Atkins, C.J., Patterson, T.L., Roppe, B.E., Kaplan, R.M. et al. (1987) Recruitment issues, health habits and the decision to participate in a health promotion programme, *Am. J. Preventive Med.* **3**, 87–94.

Beery, W., Schoenbach, V.J., Wagner, E.H., Graham, R.M. et al. (1981) *Description, analysis and assessment of health hazard/health risk appraisal programmes: final report*, National Technical Information Services, Springfield, VA.

Berkman, L.F. and Syme, S.L. (1979) Social networks, host resistance and mortality: A nine-year follow-up study of Alameda County residents, *Am. J. Epidemiol.* **109**, 186–204.

Bertera, R.L. and Cuthie, J.C. (1984) Blood pressure self-monitoring in the workplace, *J. Occup. Med.* **26**, 183–188.

Black, D.R., Coe, W.C., Friesen, J.G. and Wurtzmann, A.G. (1984) Minimal interventions for weight control: a cost-effective alternative, *Addictive Behaviour* **9**, 279–285.

Botvin, G.J. and Eng, A. (1982) The efficacy of a multicomponent approach to the prevention of cigarette smoking, *Preventive Med.* **11**, 199–211.

Broadhead, W.E., Gehlbach, S.H., DeGruy, F.V. and Kaplan, B.H. (1989) Functional versus structural social support and health care utilization in a family medicine outpatient practice, *Medical Care* **27**, 211–233.

Brownell, K.D., Cohen, R.Y., Stunkard, A.J. Felix, M.R.J. et al. (1984) Weight loss competitions at the worksite: impact on weight, moral and cost-effectiveness, *Am. J. Public Hlth.* **74**, 1283–1285.

Brownell, K.D. and Jeffery, R.W. (1987) Improving long-term weight loss: pushing the limits of treatment, *Behavioral Therapy* **18**, 353–374.

Cleary, P.E. (1984, June) *Why people take precautions against health risks.* Presented at the conference of Self-Protective Behaviour, Rutgers University.

Colon, I. (1981) Alcohol availability and cirrhosis mortality rates by gender and race, *Am. J. Public Hlth.* **71**, 1325–1328.

Cummings, K.M., Jaen, C.R. and Giovino, G. (1985) Circumstances surrounding relapse in a group of recent smokers, *Preventive Med.* **14**, 195–202.

Curry, S.J., Marlatt, G.A., Gordon, J. and Baer, J.S. (1988) A comparison of alternative theoretical approaches to smoking cessation and relapse, *Hlth Psychol.* **7**, 545–556.

Davis, A.L., Faust, R. and Ordentlich, M. (1984) Self-help smoking cessation and maintenance programmes: a comparative study with 12-month follow-up by the American Lung Association, *Am. J. Public Hlth.* **74**, 1212–1217.

Davis, K.E., Jackson, K.L., Kronenfeld, J.J. and Blair, S.N. (1987) Determinants of participation in worksite health promotion activities, *Hlth Ed. Quarterly* **17**, 18–22.

Decker, M.D., Graitcer, P.L. and Schaffner, W. (1988) Reduction in motor vehicle fatalities associated with an increase in the minimum drinking age, *J. Am. Med. Assoc.* **260**, 3604–3510.

Dielman, T.E., Shope, J.P., Leech, S.L. and Butchart, A.T. (1989) Differential effectiveness of an elementary school-based alcohol misuse prevention programme, *J. School Hlth.* **59**, 255–263.

Dwyer, T., Pierce, J.P., Hannam, C.D., and Burke, N. (1986) Evaluation of the Sydney 'Quit For Life' anti-smoking campaign: Part II, Changes in smoking prevalence, *Medical J. Australia* **144**, 344–347.

Elder, J.P., Hovell, M.F., Lasater, T.M., Wells, B.L. *et al.* (1985) Applications of behaviour modification to community health education: the case of heart disease prevention, *Hlth Ed. Quarterly* **12**, 151–169.

Ernst, N.D., Wu, M., Frommer, P., Katz, E. *et al.* (1986) Nutrition education at the point of purchase: the foods for health project evaluated, *Preventive Med.* **15**, 60–73.

Fagerstrom, K.O. (1984) Effects of nicotine chewing gum and follow-up appointments in physician-based smoking cessation, *Preventive Med.* **13**, 517–527.

Farquhar, J.W. (1978) The community-based model of lifestyle intervention trials, *Am. J. Epidemiol.* **108**, 103–111.

Farquhar, J.W., Maccoby, N., Wood, P.D., Alexander, J.K. *et al.* (1977) Community education for cardiovascular health, *Lancet* **1**, 1192–1195.

Ferguson, K.J., Yesalis, C.E., Pomrehn, P.R., and Kirkpatrick, M.B. (1989) Attitudes, knowledge, and beliefs as predictors of exercise intent and behaviour in school children, *J. School Hlth.* **59**, 112–115.

Flay, B.R. (1987) Mass media and smoking cessation: a critical review, *Am. J. Public Hlth.* **77**, 153–160.

Flay, B.R. (1986) Mass media linkages with school-based programmes for drug abuse prevention, *J. School Hlth.* **56**, 402–406.

Glasgow, R.E. and Lichtenstein, E. (1987) Long-term effects of behavioural smoking cessation interventions, *Behaviour Therapy* **18**, 297–324.

Glasgow, R.E., Schafer, L., O'Neil, H.K. (1981) Self-help books and amount of therapist contact in smoking cessation programmes, *J. Consulting and Clin. Psychol.* **46**, 659–667.

Glynn, T.J. and Manley, M.W. (1989) *How to help your patients stop smoking*, National Cancer Institute, Bethesda, MD.

Godin, G., Desharnais, R., Jobin, J., and Cook, J. (1987) The impact of physical fitness and health-age appraisal upon exercise intentions and behaviour, *J. Behavioral Med.* **10**, 241–250.

Hansen, W.B., Johnson, C.A., Flay, B.R., Graham, J.W. *et al.* (1988) Affective and social influences approaches to the prevention of multiple substance abuse among seventh grade students: results from Project SMART, *Preventive Med.* **17**, 135–154.

Harackiewicz, J.M., Sansome, C., Blair, L.W., Epstein, J.A. *et al.* (1987) Attributional processes in behaviour change and maintenance: smoking cessation and continued abstinence, *J. Consultative Clin. Psychol.* **55**, 372–378.

Heather, N., Robertson, I., McPherson, B., Allsop, S. *et al.* (1987) Effectiveness of a controlled drinking self-help manual: one-year follow-up results, *Brit. J. Clin. Psychol.* **26**, 279–287.

Hoadley, J.F., Fuchs, B.C., and Holder, H.D. (1984) The effect of alcohol beverage restrictions on consumption: a 25-year longitudinal analysis, *Am. J. Drug Alcohol Abuse* **10**, 375–401.

Holloway, R.L., Spivey, R.N., Zismer, D., and Withington, A.M. (1988) Aptitude × treatment interactions: implications for patient education research, *Hlth. Ed. Quarterly* **15**, 241–259.

Hunt, W.A. and Bespalec, D.A. (1974) An evaluation of current methods of modifying smoking behaviour, *J. Clin. Psychol.* **30**, 431–438.

Insull, W., Henderson, M., Prentice, R., Thompson, D.J. *et al.* (submitted for publication) *Results of a randomized feasibility study of a low-fat diet.*

Israel, B.A. (1985) Social networks and social support: implications for natural helper and community-level interventions, *Hlth. Ed. Quarterly* **12**, 65–80.

Iverson, D.C., Calonge, B.N., Main, D., and Holcomb, S. (1989) *BP American fitness centre evaluation: Final report*, UCHSC, Department of Family Medicine, Denver, CO.

Janz, N.K., Becker, M.H., Kirscht, J.P., Eraker, S.A. *et al.* (1987) Evaluation of a minimal-contact smoking cessation intervention in an outpatient setting, *Am. J. Public Hlth.* **77**, 805–809.

Jarvik, M.E., and Schneider, N.G. (1984) Degree of addiction and effectiveness of nicotine gum therapy for smoking, *Am. J. Psychiatry* **141**, 790–791.

Jason, L.A., Gruder, C.L., Martino, S., Flay, B.R. *et al.* (1987) Work site group meetings and the effectiveness of a televised smoking cessation intervention, *Am. J. Community Psychol.* **15**, 57–72.

Johnson, C.A., Hansen, W.B., Collins, L.M., and Graham, J.W. (1986) High school smoking prevention: results of a three-year longitudinal study, *J. Behavioral Med.* **9**, 439–452.

King, A.C., Taylor, C.B., Haskell, W.L., and Debusk, R.R. (1988) Strategies for increasing early adherence to and long-term maintenance of home-based exercise training in healthy middle-age men and women, *Am. J. Cardiology* **61**, 628–632.

Klesges, R.C., Brown, K., Pascale, R.W., Murphy, M. *et al.* (1988) Factors associated with participation, attrition and outcome in a smoking cessation programme at the workplace, *Hlth Psychol.* **7**, 575–589.

Koegel, L.K., Koegel, R.L., and Ingham, J.C. (1986) Programming rapid generalization of correct articulation through self-monitoring procedures, *J. Speech and Hearing Disorders* **51**, 24–32.

Kottke, T.E., Battista, R.N., DeFriese, G.H. and Brekke, M.L. (1987) *Attributes of successful smoking cessation interventions in medical practice: a meta-analysis of 39 controlled trials*, The Institute for the Study of Smoking Behaviour and Policy, Cambridge, MA.

Kottke, T.E., Puska, P., Salonen, J.T., Tuomilehto, J. *et al.* (1985) Projected effects of high-risk vs. population-based prevention strategies in coronary heart disease, *Am. J. Epidemiol.* **121**, 697–704.

Lando, H.A., Kalb, E.A., and McGovern, P.G. (1988) Behavioral self-help materials as an adjunct to nicotine gum, *Addictive Behaviour* **13**, 181–184.

Lane, D.S. (1983) Compliance with referrals from a cancer-screening project, *J. Family Practice* **17**, 811-817.

Lefebvre, R.C., Harden, E.A., Rakowski, W., Lasater, T.M. *et al.* (1987) Characteristics of participants in community health promotion programmes: four-year results, *Am. J. Public Hlth.* **77**, 1342–1344.

Lefebvre, R.C., Lasater, T.M., Carleton, R.A. and Peterson, G. (1987) Theory and delivery of health programming in the community: the Pawtucket Heart health programme, *Preventive Med.* **16**, 80–95.

Levenkron, J.C., and Greenland, P. (1988) Patient priorities for behavioural change: selecting from multiple coronary disease risk factors, *J. General Internal Med.* **3**, 224–229.

Lewis, B., Mann, J.I., and Mancini, M. (1986) Reducing the risk of coronary heart disease in individuals and in the population, *Lancet* **14**, 956–959.

Marburger, E.A., and Friedel, B. (1987) Seat belt legislation and seat belt effectiveness in the Federal Republic of Germany, *J. Trauma* **27**, 703–705.

Marlatt, G.A., and Gordon, J.R. (eds.) (1985) *Relapse prevention – maintenance strategies for the treatment of addictive behaviours*, Guildford Press, New York.

Mayer, J.A., Heins, J.M., Vogel, J.M., Morrison, D.C. *et al.* (1986) Promoting low-fat entrée choices in a public cafeteria, *J. Applied Behavioral Analysis* **19**, 397–402.

McLeroy, K.R., Bibeau, D., Steckler, A. and Glanz, K. (1988) An ecological perspective on health promotion programmes, *Hlth. Ed. Quarterly* **15**, 351–378.

Mechanic, D., and Cleary, P.D. (1980) Factors associated with the maintenance of positive health behaviour, *Preventive Med.* **9**, 805–814.

Millar, W.J., and Naegele, B.E. (1987) Time to quit programme, *Canadian J. Public Hlth.* **78**, 109–114.

Monahan, J.L. and Scheirer, M.A. (1988) The role of linking agents in the diffusion of health promotion programmes, *Hlth Ed. Quarterly* **15**, 417–434.

Morisky, D.E., DeMuth, N.M., Field-Fass, J., Green, L.W. *et al.* (1985) Evaluation of family health education to build social support for long-term control of high blood pressure, *Hlth. Ed. Quarterly* **12**, 35–50.

Murray, D.M. (1986) Dissemination of community health promotion programmes: the Fargo-Morehead heart health programme, *J. of School Hlth.* **56**, 375–381.

Murray, D.M., Richards, P.S., Luepker, R.V., and Johnson, C.A. (1987) The prevention of cigarettes smoking in children: two- and three-year follow-up comparisons of four prevention strategies, *J. Behavioral Med.* **10**, 595–611.

Ockene, J.K. (1987) Physician-delivered interventions for smoking cessation: strategies for increasing effectiveness, *Preventive Med.* **16**, 723–737.

Pederson, L.L., Baldwin, N. and Lefcoe, N.M. (1981) Utility of behavioural self-help manuals in a minimal-contact smoking cessation programme, *Int. J. Addiction* **16**, 1233–1239.

Pentz, M.A., Brannon, B.R., Charlin, V.L., Barrett, E.J. *et al.* (1989) The power of policy: The relationship of smoking policy to adolescent smoking, *Am. J. Public Hlth.* **79**, 857–862.

Pentz, M.A., Dwyer, J.H., MacKinnon, D.P., Flay, B.R. *et al.* (1989) A multicommunity trial for primary prevention of adolescent drug abuse: effects on drug use prevalence, *J. Am. Med. Assoc.* **261**, 3259–3266.

Perri, M.G., Lauer, J.B., Yancey, D.Z., McAdoo, W.G. *et al.* (1987) Effects of peer support and therapist contact on long-term weight loss, *J. Consultative Clin. Psychol.* **55**, 615–617.

Peterson, G., Abrams, D.B., Elder, J.P., and Beaudin, P.A. (1985) Professional vs. self-help weight loss at the worksite: the challenge of making a public health impact, *Behavioral Therapy* **16**, 213–22.

Peterson, L.R., Helgerson, S.D., Gibbons, C.M., Calhoun, C.R. *et al.* (1988) Employee smoking behaviour changes and attitudes following a restrictive policy on worksite smoking in a large company, *Public Hlth Report* **103**, 115–119.

Pierce, J.P. (1989, July) *The quitting process.* Presented at the Conference on Health Insurance and Smoking: The Future Role of Health Insurance in Promoting Smoking Cessation, Cambridge, MA.

Pierce, J.P., Dwyer, T., Frape, G., Chapman, S. *et al.* (1986) Evaluation of the Sydney 'Quit for Life' anti-smoking campaign: Part I, Achievement of intermediate goals, *Med. J. Australia* **144**, 341–344.

Pirie, P.L., Elias, W.S., Wackman, D.B., Jacobs, D.R. *et al.* (1986) Characteristics of participants and non-participants in a community cardiovascular disease risk factor screening: the Minnesota heart health programme, *Am. J. Preventive Med.* **2**, 20–25.

Prochaska, J.O. (1989, August) *What causes people to change from unhealthy to health-enhancing behaviour?* Paper presented at the American Cancer Society's Human Behaviour and Cancer Risk Reducation Conference, Bloomington, IN.

Puska, P., McAllister, A., Pekkola, J., and Koskela, K. (1981) Television in health promotion: evaluation of a national programme in Finland, *Int. J. Hlth. Ed.* **24**, 2–14.

Puska, P., Nissinen, A., Tuomilehto, J., Salonen, J.T. *et al.* (1985) The community-based strategy to prevent coronary heart disease: conclusion from the ten years of the North Karelia Project, *Ann. Rev. Public Hlth.* **6**, 147–193.

Rogers, E.M. and Shoemaker, F.F. (1971) *Communication innovations: a cross cultural approach* (2nd ed.), Free Press, New York.

Russell, M.A.H., Stapleton, J.A., Hajek, P., Jackson, P.H. (1988) District programme to reduce smoking: Can sustained intervention by general practitioners affect prevalence? *J. Epidemiol. Community Hlth.* **42**, 111–115.

Schinke, S.P., Gilchrist, L.D. and Snow, W.H. (1985) Skills intervention to prevent cigarette smoking among adolescents, *Am. J. Public Hlth.* **75**, 665–667.

Schmitz, M.F., and Fielding, J.E. (1986) Point-of-choice nutritional labelling: evaluation in a worksite cafeteria, *J. Nutritional Ed.* **18**(Supp.), S65–S68.

Seekins, T., Fawcett, S.B., Cohen, S.H., Elder, J.P. *et al.* (1988) Experimental evaluation of public policy: the case of state legislation for child passenger safety, *J. Applied Behavioral Analysis* **21**, 233–243.

Stunkard, A.J., Cohen, R.Y., and Felix, M.R.J. (1989) Weight loss competitions at the worksite: how they work and how well, *Preventive Med.* **18**, 460–474.

Vaillant, G.E. (1988) What can long-term follow-up teach us about relapse and prevention of relapse in addiction? *Brit. J. Addiction* **83**, 1147–1157.

Wagner, J.L. and Winett, R.A. (1988) Prompting one low-fat, high-fiber selection in a fast-food restaurant, *J. Applied Behavioral Analysis* **21**, 179–185.

Warner, K.E., and Murt, H.A. (1983) Premature deaths avoided by the antismokingcampaign, *Am. J. Public Hlth.* **73**, 672–677.

Zavela, K.J., Davis, L.G., Cottress, R.R. and Smith, W.E. (1988) Do only the healthy intend to participate in worksite health promotion? *Hlth. Ed. Quarterly* **15**, 259–268.

CO-ORDINATED ACTION AGAINST TOBACCO

Patti White

Introduction

Until the middle decades of this century, lung cancer was a rare disease. Alton Ochsner, one of the first people to connect the rise in cigarette smoking with the alarming increase in lung cancer deaths, was a medical student at Washington University in 1919. In that year, his professor invited him to witness an autopsy of a lung cancer patient because, he said, the condition was so rare that it was likely to be a once in a lifetime event. It was 1936 before Ochsner saw another case; that year he saw nine in six months. So struck was he by this extraordinary situation that he looked into the backgrounds of the patients: all nine were men and heavy cigarette smokers who had started smoking during the 1914–1918 war (Ochsner, 1977).

In the half-century that has elapsed since Ochsner's observation, tobacco as a cause of disease has been extensively investigated, and it is now estimated that there have been more than 57,000 technical documents published on smoking and health (USDHHS, 1989). In many countries where cigarette smoking has been common practice since the early decades of this century, tobacco is known to be the largest single, preventable cause of disease and premature death. So, as King Edward VII famously asked of tuberculosis; 'If preventable, why not prevented?'

Serious attempts to decrease smoking really began after the landmark publication of the reports of the Royal College of Physicians of London (1962) and the United States Surgeon General (1964). The initial response was to promote public education to make people, and especially children, aware of the risks. Such measures met with some success, but change was not as rapid as many had expected. There are important reasons why the problem of

decreasing tobacco use has been such an intractable one.

First, in industrialized countries, tobacco smoking is a habit practised by a large proportion of the population. For example, when the Royal College of Physicians published its first report, about half of the British adult population smoked (including 6 out of 10 men). Secondly, smoking is a habit that is socially ingrained, around which a whole set of social values has evolved; until recently, smoking was uniformly seen as a normal part of adult life. Thirdly, this image is reinforced by heavy promotion; cigarettes are among the most extensively advertised consumer products. Moreover, there are strong commercial interests that resist attempts by public authorities to limit the freedom of the tobacco industry to promote and sell its products. Finally, the product that is being sold as a promoter of friendship, a badge of adulthood and sophistication, is highly addictive. The story of tobacco control at the close of the 20th century will be seen as a novel project to affect a wide-scale change in attitudes and behaviours towards this uniquely dangerous product.

Tobacco as a cause of cancer

Scope of the tobacco pandemic

The World Health Organization has declared that Europe, as the rest of the world, is in the steeply increasing phase of a huge pandemic of immense size (WHO, 1990). It has been estimated that by the mid-1980s tobacco caused about 800,000 deaths per year in the countries that comprise the WHO's European Region. About half of those deaths were attributable to cancer.

British epidemiologist Richard Peto has estimated that on present trends, 100 million of the 850 million people now alive in Europe are likely to be killed by tobacco. The number of deaths will escalate in the next century. By the year 2025, tobacco will have caused the deaths of about two million Europeans annually; the worldwide annual total will be about eight million people. In the second quarter of the next century, mortality from tobacco may be about 10 million a year if present patterns persist. About half of these deaths will occur in middle age (40 to 69 years) resulting in a considerable loss of life expectancy (Peto, 1988).

The vastness of these numbers makes them almost incomprehensible, but they represent the lives of people who are already alive – today's children. The reality is that these figures are likely to be too conservative. They are estimates of the deaths attributable to tobacco if consumption follows its present pattern. Although per capita cigarette consumption shows little growth in developed countries and is falling in some, it continues to rise sharply in developing countries (FAO, 1989).

Cancer deaths from tobacco

Tobacco has become responsible for one in three cancer deaths in some countries (Doll and Peto, 1981). Richard Peto has estimated that by the mid-1980s, of the 840,000 annual male cancer deaths in Europe, 360,000 could have been attributed to tobacco. Annual cancer deaths attributable to tobacco during the same period for European females was 40,000 (Peto, 1988).

Lung cancer

Lung cancer, the type of cancer most closely associated with tobacco smoking, is believed to be the most common fatal cancer in the world today and its incidence is increasing rapidly (IARC, 1988). The International Agency for Research on Cancer (IARC) has said that tobacco smoking causes most cases of lung cancer and it accounts for 80% (and more

than 90% in men) of this disease in populations where widespread cigarette smoking has been practised for two generations or more (IARC, 1988). Even larger proportions obtain in some countries, such as Britain, where over 95% of lung cancer in men has been attributed to this cause (Doll, 1988).

Other cancers

Tobacco smoking is an important cause of cancers of the mouth, pharynx, larynx and oesophagus in both men and women, and the risk increases with greater tobacco consumption (USDHHS, 1989). Smoking also appears to be an important cause of pancreatic cancer, with mortality ratios for cigarette smokers some two to three times higher than for non-smokers (USDHHS, 1989). Cancers of the lower urinary tract, specifically the bladder and renal pelvis, have been consistently associated with cigarette smoking and several studies have shown an association between cancer of the kidney and cigarette smoking (IARC, 1988).

Evidence has accumulated in the past few years that indicates that a number of other cancers should be added to the list of those caused by smoking: cancer of the stomach, cervix uteri, liver, nasal sinuses and leukaemia (Doll, 1988).

Cancers caused by use of oral ('smokeless') tobacco

In the Western hemisphere, use of tobacco in the form of chewing tobacco or snuff was overtaken by cigarette smoking in the middle of this century, although oral tobacco is still used widely in the Indian subcontinent, south-east Asia and parts of the middle east. Use of oral snuff in Europe is largely confined to the Scandinavian countries where increased promotion and clever marketing in recent years have revived the habit and sold it to a larger, younger audience (Nordgrun and Ramstron, 1990).

Smokeless tobacco use has been associated with an increased risk of cancer of the mouth in epidemiological studies carried out in Europe and North America. In Asia, the habit of using chewing tobacco with lime or with betel quid (a mixture of betel leaf and areca nut) has been associated with increased risk for oral cancer (IARC, 1988).

Lung cancer from passive smoking

Before the 1980s, breathing other people's smoke was thought of primarily as a nuisance rather than a health hazard. While some scientists thought it plausible that even low levels of exposure to the carcinogens in tobacco smoke might be dangerous, the harmful effects of passive smoking were believed to be confined to vulnerable groups, such as infants and small children and people with other health problems, such as asthma. Expert scientific committees in Britain, Australia, the United States as well as IARC have reviewed the growing body of scientific and medical evidence that has emerged over the past decade and all have concluded that environmental tobacco smoke should be considered a public health problem.

In Britain, the Government's expert advisory body, the Independent Scientific Committee on Smoking and Health, has estimated that non-smokers exposed to environmental tobacco smoke have a 10 to 30% increased risk of lung cancer. The Committee's fourth report, published in 1988, explained that this: '… might amount to several hundred out of the current annual total of about 40,000 lung cancer deaths in the United Kingdom, a small but not negligible proportion' (ISCSH, 1988).

Although the risk of lung cancer from passive smoking is small, it is not insignificant when compared to other cancer risks. It has been estimated that the risk of lung cancer from passive smoking is some 50 to 100 times greater than that from exposure to chrysotile asbestos, normally found in asbestos-containing buildings (Peto and Doll, 1986). It is true that non-smokers' risk of contracting lung cancer through passive smoking is much less than that which smokers experience through active smoking, but in principle, hazards to which we are involuntarily exposed should be much smaller than those which we undertake voluntarily.

Controlling the tobacco pandemic

Every European country has taken steps to try to reduce tobacco consumption. While many of these initiatives have been excellent in themselves, they have not proved sufficient to bring about the necessary decreases in tobacco consumption or to keep new generations from taking up the habit. Since the early days of public information campaigns about smoking, it has become clear that imparting knowledge to the public is not enough. Along with other areas of public health, the anti-tobacco campaign has developed a different understanding of what it is to promote health. Public policies that make healthier choices easier choices, and new ways of working that co-ordinate action and build alliances between local, national and international statutory and voluntary bodies are necessary for progress on a variety of issues. Because tobacco use is so firmly socially and economically entrenched in European countries, and tobacco related deaths so very common, people working in tobacco control have also increasingly recognized that they must also act as 'advocates' for health in order to challenge the widespread acceptance of smoking.

'Advocacy' generally refers to those efforts to shape opinion in support of public policy initiatives, usually by utilizing the mass media. As distinct from lobbying, which is an attempt to influence legislators, the objective of advocacy is to shift public attitudes and perceptions. This may be either in a positive way, by raising public awareness and developing a consensus in favour of the advocated policy, (for example, by arguing for cleaner, smoke-free public environments) or negatively, as a force of opposition to statements that are misleading and contrary to public health interests, such as countering tobacco industry claims that advertising bans do not affect children's smoking. Both advocacy and lobbying recognize that smoking is not an individual choice but a political, health, social and economic issue.

A comprehensive tobacco policy

It has long been recognized that it is necessary for countries to adopt comprehensive tobacco policies if they wish to lessen their burden of smoking-related deaths and diseases. Such an approach has the enthusiastic endorsement of the World Health Organization, the International Union Against Cancer and other expert bodies. At the same time, it is clear that tobacco use is not just a national problem and international co-operation and collaboration are increasingly sought as a way to find appropriate solutions. Nowhere is this more evident than within the European Community.

The main components of a tobacco-control programme can be seen as achieving certain broad objectives, although some policies will fall into more than one category. There are those policies that prevent tobacco use by trying to make an individual's decision not to smoke the easier option. These include policies on tobacco price and taxation; limiting availability of tobacco products, for example, bans on sales to minors or forbidding the sale of new tobacco products, such as oral tobacco; ensuring public places such as schools, transport, health premises and the workplace are smoke-free; promoting public information and education including health warnings on tobacco packs.

Other policies are aimed at current smokers. These might include health education and information to encourage smokers to attempt to quit; smoking cessation research and services; or modifying the toxic emissions of cigarettes for those smokers who are unable to stop.

Still other policy initiatives affect the social acceptability of smoking. Measures such as

banning tobacco advertising and sponsorship and ensuring that public places are smoke-free are now thought to be among the most important components of a tobacco-control policy.

Many of these policy areas are already being affected by European Community Directives and the move towards a single European market in 1992 will ensure that decisions about national tobacco policies will be taken in Brussels.

Labelling

The most important change in tobacco labelling in Europe was the adoption, in 1989, by the EC Council of Ministers of a Directive to standardize health warnings. From January 1992, all tobacco products must carry the message, 'tobacco seriously damages your health' on the front of the packet in the language of the country in which it is being sold. A second warning from an approved list must appear on the second large surface. Tobacco packs must also state the nicotine and tar yields.

The United Kingdom was the only Member state to oppose this Directive and its passage has far-reaching consequences for the country. The United Kingdom has previously relied on self-regulation by the tobacco industry, through a series of so-called 'voluntary agreements', to control tobacco advertising, sponsorship, tar levels and labelling. Many countries, such as Canada and New Zealand, which had allowed the tobacco companies to be similarly self-regulating have abandoned that in favour of legislation. These countries, and critics of the British system, argue that voluntary agreements are inadequate because they are industry-led policy instruments with no system of ensuring compliance and no penalties for abuse.

Tar yields

Another EC Directive requires that by the end of 1992, cigarettes sold in Community countries should have a maximum tar yield of

15 mg per cigarette. By 1998, this should be a 12 mg maximum.

Tobacco price

'Every tobacco price decision is also a health policy decision', is how the government of Finland was advised to consider taxation policy by its National Board of Health. The price of tobacco is considered to be a crucial element in any tobacco-control strategy. Crudely put, the demand for cigarettes varies inversely with price: when tobacco becomes cheaper, consumption goes up, when it becomes more expensive, the opposite result is achieved. For this reason, governments are under pressure from health authorities to increase the price of tobacco to at least keep pace with inflation. This is also thought to be an important strategy for preventing smoking among young people as adolescents are more sensitive than adults to price rises.

EC tax harmonization

Tobacco prices vary markedly within the EC; there is about a six-fold difference in cigarette prices throughout Europe (Townsend, 1988). As a consequence of the Single European Act, the European Commission has proposed a set of minimum and maximum rates of tax to be levied on tobacco and alcohol in order to harmonize taxation in 1992. If implemented, these proposals would have the effect of raising tobacco taxes significantly in some countries but lowering them in others, such as Denmark, Ireland and the United Kingdom. There is concern in these countries that harmonization will result in increased tobacco consumption. In 1988, the Chancellor of the Exchequer of the United Kingdom requested that tobacco and alcohol be exempted from harmonization on health grounds, but no compromise had been reached at the time of writing.

Tobacco advertising and sponsorship

The tobacco industry opposes attempts to curb tobacco promotion more fiercely than any other area of tobacco control. This has led many people working to promote health to conjecture that the industry sees promotion as its prime avenue for ensuring public acceptability of its products and creating a new generation of smokers. There is a growing body of evidence to indicate that children learn to recognize and decipher tobacco advertisements at a surprisingly early age and that approval of advertising is a predictor of later smoking. The government of New Zealand recently reviewed the evidence from 18 countries and concluded that legislation to ban promotion was related to decreases in uptake of smoking by young people. This review also concluded that partial bans were not effective because tobacco advertising budgets were diverted to different avenues of promotion as others became blocked (Toxic Substances Board, 1989).

Thus far Member States have not been able to agree on initiatives to limit tobacco advertising and sponsorship within the EC. Four Member States explicitly support a complete ban while seven others have indicated support. Germany, the United Kingdom and the Netherlands are opposed to any ban.

As a result of the Directive on Broadcasting in the Community, tobacco advertisements will be banned from radio and television. Bans on broadcast advertising are common but the Directive will cause some changes in national regulations. For example, although cigarette advertisements have been banned in United Kingdom broadcast media since 1965, the new Directive will extend this ban to all tobacco products; cigar and pipe tobacco advertising will disappear from British television.

Challenges for the 1990s

Clearing the air – creating a smoke-free environment

The demand for no-smoking accommodation in public areas is not a new phenomenon. In the United Kingdom, the Royal College of

Physicians' third report on tobacco, *Smoking or Health* (1977), indicated that seven out of 10 British adults responding to a 1976 survey said they favoured greater restrictions on smoking in hospitals, restaurants, cinemas, buses and aeroplanes.

Throughout the 1980s, public pressure for more smoke-free spaces increased in many countries. By 1987, over three-quarters (77%) of those interviewed in a European Community survey were in favour of restricting smoking in public places. Several factors influenced this change, but by far the most important was the appearance of greater medical and scientific evidence on passive smoking. This information legitimized non-smokers' desire to be free from the nuisance and discomfort of tobacco smoke. The response of public authorities has been either to seek voluntary change or to pursue legislative means to guarantee the right of non-smokers to smoke-free air.

Smoking in public places and the European Community

In May 1989, the EC Council of Health Ministers reached an agreement on a 'mixed' resolution to ban smoking in enclosed public places. This mean that Member States could ban smoking in schools, hospitals, public transport and so on by legislation or by 'other means'. The resolution specified that dedicated zones could be reserved for smokers, but in the event of a conflict, the rights of non-smokers should take precedence. The Member States have agreed to report every two years on the progress of implementation of the resolution with the understanding that if sufficient progress is not made, legislation will be pursued.

European Community countries have responded differently to this resolution. The United Kingdom has chosen not to legislate, but to seek voluntary change. Ireland, on the other hand, has made the Tobacco (Health Promotion and Protection) Regulation 1990 under powers conferred on the Minister of Health by the Tobacco (Health Promotion and Protection) Act, 1988. The Regulation designates areas where smoking is prohibited, including state offices and public buildings, and others where it is restricted, such as hospitals. The Irish Government unambiguously acknowledges that the guarantee of smoke-free air is a central plank of its effort to control smoking.

> The Act is considered crucial in the Government's strategy to reduce tobacco consumption. The social approbation for non-smoking is growing in Ireland and this Act is designed to accelerate this by developing an environment that is hostile to smoking and conducive to non-smoking and good health.
>
> (Lyons, 1990)

The resolution has acted as a trigger for other community countries to take action. In May 1990, Belgium adopted a Royal Decree to strengthen its already extensive legislation restricting smoking. The Netherlands legislated to restrict smoking in government buildings or those controlled by government-supported organizations. The French National Assembly also adopted wide-ranging tobacco legislation in 1990 which included smoking restrictions in public places.

Smoking in the workplace

Exposure to environmental tobacco smoke at work is a particular problem because of the long hours spent in the workplace. Considering that many people have a working life of 40 years or longer, a lifetime's exposure to smoking at work can be substantial. Opinion surveys show that an increasing number of people believe that employees have a right to work in smoke-free air. A 1987 National Opinion Polls survey in the United Kingdom reported that 85% of those interviewed thought that passive smoking was a health hazard and that 86% thought that non-smokers had the right to work in air free of tobacco smoke (Marsh and Matheson, 1983; Hughes-Onslow, 1987).

Having a no-smoking policy for the workplace is becoming increasingly popular both in countries with legislation that bans smoking at work and in those with no legal protection for non-smokers in the workplace. The value of having a formal, written policy is that it not only protects the right of employees to clean air at work but also provides an avenue for resolving any possible conflicts which might arise between non-smokers who want to enjoy this right and smokers who will have to surrender some of their accustomed privileges.

Experience in North America and Australia as well as parts of Europe shows the importance of negotiated agreements to secure harmonious change. Important elements of policy formulation are: informing staff members of the effects on health of environmental tobacco smoke; determining what the wishes of the majority of the workforce are; publicizing the proposed changes and encouraging discussion; providing encouragement and support for those employees who wish to stop smoking. A workplace no-smoking policy is a health-promotion exercise for non-smokers and smokers alike: while protecting non-smokers, the policy ensures that smokers will cut down their consumption and some will be encouraged to quit.

Creating a smoke-free Health Service

Health premises have been a primary focus of action to create a smoke-free environment. Such premises should be healthy environments for patients and health workers alike. There is also a common sentiment that health premises are the flagship of smoke-free spaces and that health workers have little justification in promoting tobacco control before they put their own house in order.

Women and smoking

Cigarette smoking became socially acceptable for women in many countries about the time of the Second World War. The big increases in cigarette smoking then are now reflected in the rising rates of female lung cancer. Great Britain has one of the world's highest female lung cancer death rates and in Scotland the disease has already overtaken breast cancer as the leading form of cancer death in women (OPCS, 1987).

Now, in much of Europe, the number of female smokers is reaching parity with that of males. This 'equality' is especially marked among the young. According to Europe Against Cancer data, smoking prevalence among young European women (39%) is about the same as that among young men (EC, 1987). The trend can also be seen among children and adolescents. The WHO Cross National Survey of Children's Health found only a small difference in girls' and boys' smoking with more girls than boys smoking in some countries (Nutbeam *et al.*, 1988).

Tapping the market

Since the 1970s, cigarette manufacturers have been nurturing the women's market with cigarette brands and advertisements targeted specifically at women. In 1976, Philip Morris attempted a United Kingdom launch of 'Virginia Slims', a brand which had been marketed very successfully in the United States with a slogan ('You've come a long way, baby') that traded on women's growing desire for economic, civil and social equality. The brand never attained the degree of popularity in Britain that it enjoyed across the Atlantic, but other 'women's' brands, such as 'Vogue' and 'Kim', which are widely marketed in Europe, have also attempted to tap this market.

Cigarette brands designed to appeal to women are often sold by an appeal to their 'feminine' attributes and are often advertised with reference to their lightness, elegance or slimness. Perhaps this is in lieu of the specific claims of early advertising, like that for Lucky Strike which, appealing to women's use of smoking to control weight, abjured women 'to keep a slender figure – reach for a Lucky instead of a sweet'.

Faced with advertising restrictions that have made it increasingly difficult to create advertisements especially aimed at women, cigarette manufacturers have turned increasingly to advertising in magazines read almost exclusively by women. A survey of 60 European women's magazines found that tobacco advertising was extensive in this medium and that editors generally accepted cigarette advertisements except when forbidden to do so by national regulations (Amos, 1990).

An increasing number of women's magazines are published in different editions in several European countries. Variations not only in national advertising regulations but also in attitudes to tobacco are reflected in the different editions. For example, the English language versions of magazines such as *Vogue*, *Elle* or *Marie Claire* do not accept cigarette ads and have a policy of not showing models smoking in editorial or fashion pages (Amos *et al.*, 1991). The Spanish and French versions of the same magazine often portray fashion models smoking accompanied by scenes and text that convey a sense of power, seductiveness or luxury: 'douce heure en short rose volupté' (an intimate moment in the voluptuousness of pink shorts) *Elle* (Comité Français d'Education pour la Santé, 1989). As trade and cultural barriers in Europe disappear, it is likely that the influence of European women's magazines will increase.

Less developed countries

Although the tobacco industry is far from losing money in developed countries, the downturn in consumption in its traditional, most profitable markets has given the industry a taste of the future. These companies now look toward the huge potential market of the developing world, not to mention the newly available markets of Central and Eastern Europe. The lucrative Asian market in particular has made the U.S. tobacco manufacturers, according to one tobacco trade magazine, 'wring their hands in anticipation

and pat their wallets with hope' (*Tobacco Reporter*, 1987).

One major attraction of the developing world is that even if individuals are too poor to smoke heavily, the sheer number of consumers equals profitability for the tobacco manufacturers. These populous countries already have huge numbers of smokers. China alone smoked nearly 29% of the total world consumption of cigarettes in 1988 (Chapman and Wong, 1990). Moreover, the population of much of the developing world is growing at a more rapid rate than that in more industrialized countries, thus increasing the attractiveness of this market for tobacco manufacturers.

Selling smoke

Unfettered by the marketing restrictions under which they have been forced to operate in industrialized countries, tobacco manufacturers have a free hand to promote smoking in much of the developing world. In many advertisements smoking is quite blatantly associated with sophistication, western cosmopolitan lifestyles and material wealth. Many people find shocking the difference between the fantasy aspirations presented by these advertisements and the powerlessness and poverty that is the reality of the customers' lives.

Smoking is not common among women in the Third World. For the tobacco industry, this also represents a market of great potential and moves are already afoot to exploit it. In India, brands such as 'Charm' are targeted at the young and another, 'Ms', is aimed at upwardly mobile young women. The advertisements for 'Ms' show a powerful picture of a modern, young Indian woman wearing Western clothes rather than the traditional sari. Critics have accused the tobacco company of trying to co-opt young women's aspirations to independence and freedom from cultural pressures in order to create a market for cigarettes where none currently exists (Crossette, 1990).

Adding to the burden of the Third World

As creation of new markets for cigarettes will bring profit to the transnational tobacco companies, it will bring an additional burden of illness to countries and health services which still have pressing problems with malnutrition and infectious diseases. In some cases, the epidemic has already arrived: by 1985, the World Health Organization had already named tobacco as the leading cause of death in Brazil (*New Scientist*, 1985). But for most developing countries, the problems caused by tobacco are more immediate than the diseases that will appear in 20 years' time. There is an existing economic burden: although some developing countries make money from growing and exporting tobacco, the majority have a large deficit balance of trade in tobacco and import far more than they produce or export (Chapman and Wong, 1990). Even more pressing for some countries is the environmental burden posed by the effects of deforestation, the most serious environmental problem facing the developing world.

Tobacco curing requires an extraordinary amount of energy. While gas or oil is used in industrialized countries, these sources of energy are too expensive for many developing countries which use firewood instead. For every 300 cigarettes made in these circumstances, a tree is burned. That means that for each acre of tobacco flue-cured by wood, an acre of woodland disappears (Muller, 1978). Although the amount of wood used in tobacco production is small compared to total consumption of wood in tobacco-growing countries, a high proportion of these tobacco-growing areas are in parts of the world identified by the United Nations' Food and Agriculture Organization as being in 'wood deficit or prospective wood deficit situations (FAO, 1989).

European Community tobacco subsidies

Problems of the world economy and environment are everyone's concern, but Europeans have a special interest. Not only are three of the world's seven large transnational tobacco companies registered in Europe, but European Community policies are contributing to the health problems of developing countries.

Through the Common Agricultural Policy, the EC subsidizes tobacco growing in Europe by about 1138.8 million ecu per annum; that is about £2 million per day. (By contrast, the Europe Against Cancer programme receives 9 million ecu per annum, or just under £16,000 per day) (*Lancet*, 1990). This policy has been warmly criticized not only because of the health implications but also because the subsidy policy is economically flawed.

Although intended to give financial security to European farmers, the real outcome of the subsidy during the last decade has been to increase the number of European countries where tobacco is grown, to increase the amount of tobacco being produced and to increase the amount of public money paid out in tobacco subsidies. Most of the tobacco produced is of a high-tar variety that is not to European taste and about 70% of the tobacco consumed here is imported. Thus the European 'tobacco mountain' has quadrupled in the past decade. About 40% of the unwanted, high-tar tobacco grown with EC support is exported, often at low, 'dumping' prices. Critics claim that through this policy the EC is exacerbating health and balance of payment problems in developing countries. Meanwhile, only the British and Belgian governments currently support a reduction of CAP subsidies for tobacco production.

References

Amos, A. (1990) *Women's magazines and tobacco: the preliminary findings of a survey on the tobacco policies of the top women's magazines in Europe*, Proceedings of the 7th World Conference on Tobacco and Health, Perth, Australia, (in press).

Amos, A., Jacobson, B. and White, P. (1991) Cigarette advertising policy and coverage of smoking and health in British women's magazines, *Lancet* **337**, 93–96.

Brazil tops third world league for deaths from smoking (1985) *New Scientist*, 14 February, cited in Chapman and Wong, 1990.

Chapman, S. and Wong. W.L. (1990) *Tobacco control in the Third World: a resource atlas*, International Organization of Consumers Unions, Penang, Malaysia.

Comité Français d'Education pour la Santé (1989) *Le tabac dans la press feminine en 1988*, Paris.

Commission des Communautés Européennes, l'Europe contre le Cancer (1987) *Les Européennes et la prévention du cancer. Une étude d'opinion public*, Bruxelles.

Crossette, B. (1990) New cigarette sparks a furore in India, *International Herald Tribune*, 19th March.

Doll, R. (1988) *Tobacco related disease*. Paper presented to the First European Conference on Tobacco Policy, Madrid, 7–11 November 1988.

Doll, R. and Peto, R. (1981) *The causes of cancer*, Oxford University Press. Oxford.

Europe against for cancer, *Lancet* **336**, 1036.

Food and Agriculture Organization of the United Nations (1989) *The economic significance of tobacco*. FAO Economic and Social Development Paper 85, Rome.

Hughes-Onslow, J. (1987) Office smokers losing battle, (London) *Evening Standard*, 27th July 1987.

Independent Scientific Committee on Smoking and Health (1988) *Fourth Report of the Independent Scientific Committee on Smoking and Health*, HMSO, London.

International Agency for Research on Cancer (1988) *Tobacco or health? Smoke-free Europe Series: 4.* World Health Organization Regional Office for Europe/International Agency for Research on Cancer/Europe Against Cancer, Copenhagen.

Lyons, M. (1990) *Tobacco legislation in Ireland; an overview*, Public Health Division, Department of Health, Dublin.

Marsh, A. and Matheson, J. (1983) *Smoking attitudes and behaviours*, HMSO, London.

Muller, M. (1978) *Tobacco and the Third World: tomorrow's epidemic?* War on Want, London.

Nordgrun, P. and Ramstron, L. (1990) Moist snuff in Sweden – tradition and evolution, *Br. J. of Addiction* **85**, 1107–1112.

Nutbeam, D., Mendoza, R. and Newman, R. (1988) *Planning for a smoke-free generation*, Smoke-free Europe Series: 6. World Health Organization Regional Office for Europe/Europe Against Cancer, Copenhagen.

Ochsner, A. (1977) *Proceedings of the 3rd World Conference on Smoking and Health*, U.S. Department of Health, Education and Welfare. Washington, DC.

Office of Populations Censuses and Surveys (1987) *Deaths by cause*, OPCS London, and General Registrar Office, Edinburgh.

Peto, J. and Doll, R. (1986) Passive smoking, *Br. J. Cancer* **54**, 381–383.

Peto, R. (1988) *The future effects caused by smoking*, a presentation made to the First European Conference on Tobacco Policy, Madrid, 7-11 November 1988.

Royal College of Physicians (1977) *Smoking or health: the third report of the Royal College of Physicians of London*, Pitman Medical, Tunbridge Wells.

Tobacco Reporter 1987, 114, **8**, 34.

Townsend, J. (1988) *Tobacco price and the smoking epidemic*, Smoke-free Europe Series: 9. World Health Organization Regional Office for Europe/Europe against Cancer, Copenhagen.

Toxic Substances Board (1989) *Health or tobacco: an end to tobacco advertising and promotion*, Department of Health, Wellington.

US Department of Health and Human Services (1989) *Reducing the health consequences of smoking: 25 years of progress. A report of the Surgeon General*, Office on Smoking and Health DHHS Publication No. (CDC) 89-8411, Rockville, MD.

World Health Organization Regional Office for Europe (1990). *It can be done: a smoke-free Europe; report of the First European Conference on Tobacco Policy*, WHO Regional Publications, European Series No.30. Copenhagen.

FOOD POLICY AND CANCERS

Verner Wheelock

Introduction

It is now becoming clear from research in many different fields that there is a relationship between habitual diet and the development of the degenerative diseases, which include certain cancers and diseases of the heart and arteries. Recommendations for the public on what constitutes a healthy diet are being formulated by official government bodies. This information is becoming widely available with the result that there is growing interest among health professionals and food consumers. Various attempts are being made to promote the concept of healthy eating.

However, it is crucial to recognize that the choice of diet and food intake by an individual is influenced and constrained by a number of factors.

Physiological

To function effectively the body must have a diet containing all those nutrients known to be essential for normal existence. Much of our knowledge on nutritional requirements was developed before World War II and the lessons of the research findings were incorporated into the war-time system of food control. A significant improvement in public health resulted, because much disability prior to World War II was caused by nutritional deficiencies.

Although we have a comprehensive knowledge of those nutrients which are essential, it is much more difficult to determine the optimum amount of nutrients that should be consumed. A fundamental problem is that there can be very wide differences between individuals in their actual requirements. There is plenty of reliable evidence to show that individuals on precisely the same food intake respond quite differently. For example, one person can remain at the same weight, while another can get fat very quickly. Individual nutrient requirements are influenced by a variety of factors including other constituents in the diet, stage of growth, and basal metabolic rate (the body's idling speed). Additional requirements are needed for heavy exercise, pregnancy and lactation.

Psychological

In affluent societies, most people eat only those foods they like and enjoy. Taste, appearance, texture and smell all help to influence a person's choice of food. Nevertheless, an individual's appreciation of these characteristics is not fixed and can therefore be changed. Those who regularly take sugar in their tea or coffee become conditioned to the sweet taste and so find the unsweetened beverage unpleasant. But if they take the conscious decision to persist without sugar, they soon adapt to the new taste. If motivation to change is strong, possibly for health reasons, the reconditioning process can occur very rapidly.

Economic

Clearly, the relationship between price and income does have a strong influence on food choice. As income rises, there is normally an increase in the amount of money spent on food. Since there is a physical limit to the amount of food that can actually be consumed, the tendency is to increase the amounts of expensive foods in the diet and decrease consumption of the cheaper foods. Hence the almost universal increase in the proportion of animal products consumed as living standards improve.

A characteristic example of how economic factors influence choice of food is shown by sales of butter and margarine in Britain during the 1950s and 1960s. At that time, a change in the price of one would result in a shift in demand from one to the other that was quite predictable.

Functional

Much of contemporary housework is associated with food. Shopping, storage, preparation, cooking, serving and clearing up after meals can require considerable time and effort. To some extent, the actual amount and type of work is determined by the nature of the meals being prepared, which, in turn, has a bearing on the food selected. The growth of convenience food markets is a clear indication that consumers are prepared to pay the extra cost in order to reduce the amount of time and effort associated with home preparation of meals.

The growth of car ownership has been a crucial factor in the development of supermarkets because it provides shoppers with the means to transport a large quantity of goods. It is much more difficult to take home several bags of food using public transport, especially if accompanied by young children!

Cultural

Attitudes towards certain food items are often deeply embedded in the cultural norms of society. Acceptability can vary between countries, between social classes and between religious groups. Similarly, ideas on meal structure and cooking practice vary from one culture to another. Views on acceptability can also change with time.

Individual attitudes and beliefs

As a general rule, people will not eat anything they regard as poisonous, or they believe will be hazardous to their health. Personal beliefs

on which foods are *healthy* or not and how much of each food should be eaten, exert a powerful influence on choice of food. Personal belief is particularly crucial where categoric scientific evidence is lacking or where public understanding of nutritional issues is poor.

In a peasant society, the availability of a range of food is often quite restricted and the actual diet can be largely determined by what will grow in the locality. In those circumstances, the prime concern of governments is to maintain an adequate supply of food within the context of what is culturally acceptable, although it should be recognized that, in an emergency, deeply held taboos may be overcome if the alternative is starvation. Nevertheless, there can be considerable resistance to strange foods. For example, in certain developing countries, some aspects of the Green Revolution failed: the indigenous population refused to accept products of newly introduced species because the characteristics were different from those of the native ones.

Recent changes in food consumption patterns

Since World War II, there have been major changes in what people actually eat.

First, living standards throughout Europe have continued to improve so that the proportion of income spent on food has decreased. In Britain today, it is now about 14%, although another 6% or so is spent on food that is eaten outside the home. This means that price is now much less important than it used to be. For example, in Britain in recent years, the consumption of eggs has fallen even though real prices have decreased. Similarly, there has been an increase in fruit consumption despite the fact that the price has increased in real terms. However, it should also be emphasized that those who have low incomes, such as the unemployed and single-parent families, may spend 50% or more of their income on food. For those people, price of food is paramount.

Second, the increase in the proportion of married women at work has had a profound impact on food patterns. Because of pressure on time to do the necessary preparation, there has been a growth in demand for convenience foods such as fish fingers and pizzas. More recently, there has been a demand for complete ready meals.

Third, there is now an enormous range of foods from which to choose. This means that consumers can select products which they feel match up to their own special requirements.

The role of the multiple retailers

The most significant phenomenon in the modern food chain to have occurred since World War II is the growth of multiple retailers. In many European countries, small food shops have been replaced with large modern superstores which enable the shopper to obtain all the food required on a single visit. These stores usually provide a very large number of food products – in the order of 15–20,000 – which means that for each group of foods, many different varieties are on offer.

The food retailing scene in Britain has a number of characteristics that are worth explaining. First, there is a high degree of concentration; in 1989, 52% of all food was purchased from just four companies.

Second, there is very heavy emphasis on private brands. These are products which are formulated by specialists, such as food technologists and home economists, employed by the retailers. This approach was pioneered by Marks & Spencer who lead the way in terms of quality, technical standards and profitability.

Third, buying and distribution has been centralized. Each national chain of supermarkets has four to six depots in different parts of the country. Almost all of the food from the suppliers is delivered to these depots and then despatched from here to the stores. This is only possible because of the existence of a national motorway system.

The net effect of all this is a shift in the balance of power within the food chain in favour of the consumers and retailers at the expense of the manufacturers and farmers. It is especially important to note that consumers do now have very considerable influence because of the competition between the retailers to keep in tune with what consumers want.

On the Continent, there has also been a growth of multiple retailers, especially in France, Germany, Belgium, Holland and Denmark, but there is, as yet, very little centralized buying and distribution. For example, in France, much of the buying is actually done locally and the retail multiples do not have the staff and equipment necessary for centralized buying. Furthermore, the tolls on motorways would add to the costs. Nevertheless, there are indications that some of the French retailers are showing interest in this approach. Certainly there is considerable interest from Continental Europe in what the British retailers are doing because profit margins in Britain are about three times higher.

Because the buying power of these retailers is so big and they control such a large share of the total market, they can virtually dictate terms to their suppliers. Since they are not 'locked in' to specific processes linked to expensive equipment, it is very easy for them to alter their range – all they have to do is switch suppliers. By contrast, manufacturers may find it difficult and expensive to alter their products. As a consequence, the retailers have little difficulty in responding to changes in demand by their consumers. Most of the major retailers now have large technical departments, which are responsible for 'own label' products that now constitute about 50% of all food products on the supermarket shelves.

Therefore, using their own resources, these retailers can and do formulate the specifications for new products in the light of contemporary consumer interests, attitude and concerns. Furthermore, the specialists ensure that the suppliers do follow the agreed instructions on how the foods should be produced.

Factors influencing the contemporary consumer

With this background, it is particularly relevant to examine how consumers are influenced in their attitudes to and purchase behaviour towards food. There is no doubt that many people are prepared to pay high prices for quality food. However, during the last 10 years, it has become evident that health factors are of importance to consumers.

Nowadays, the real killers are the degenerative diseases, such as coronary heart disease, diabetes and many forms of cancer. Scientific research has now produced evidence to suggest that diet does play a key role in the development of these conditions. Furthermore, it is evident that the public is becoming aware of some of the potential links between diet and disease. Unfortunately, there is widespread confusion amongst consumers about the relationship between food and health. Hence it is worthwhile examining how and why the messages get through to the public.

The starting point is invariably some kind of scientific research. I choose the term 'scientific research' carefully because some extremely dubious claims can be lumped together with bona fide investigations, and the public may have no way of distinguishing between the two.

With some of the research, the results are pretty well definitive so that the policy is quite obvious and can be implemented without controversy. A good example of this is the legislation requiring margarine to be fortified with vitamin D in order to prevent rickets.

On the other hand, it is very much more difficult with the degenerative diseases. Usually these are multi-factorial so the role of the food has to be linked in with other causes. Furthermore, there is usually a long time span between cause and effect. For example, there can be a 20 to 30-year gap between exposure to a carcinogenic agent and the disease actually manifesting itself. Therefore, experimental investigations can be extremely prolonged and, in any case, it is not usually possible to conduct them on humans. As a consequence, there has to be a fairly heavy reliance on epidemiological investigations. Hence trying to establish the relationship between diet and the different degenerative diseases is extremely difficult and progress is fairly slow.

The real world is rather different. There are demands for answers and recommendations from pressure groups, from governments and from the media. Anyone is free to read the scientific journals with papers describing current work and draw their own conclusions. Commercial interests are continually looking out for scientific findings which can be used to market food products. This kind of thing is, of course, extremely unhelpful to the consumer because the consumer is at the receiving end of a variety of messages devised by people with varying degrees of interest and competence.

In an attempt to introduce order into this kind of chaos, governments and other official bodies often set up a committee given a brief to evaluate the current state of scientific knowledge on the topic or issue and make recommendations for policy based on their findings.

In Britain, the National Advisory Committee on Nutrition Education (NACNE) was constituted in 1978 with the brief to bring nutrition education up to date. Very early on, it recognized that it would not be able to progress until it had some guidelines on what actually constituted a healthy diet. As a result, the Committee asked Professor Philip James to assemble a group and prepare the guidelines. Eventually the report of the group was published with the recommendations shown in Table 1.

Table 1 Summary of NACNE recommendations

	Base line	Short term	Long term
Total fat, % energy	38	34	30
Saturated fat, % energy	18	15	10
Polyunsaturated fat, % energy	4	5	?
P/S ratio	0.24	0.32	?
Sugar, % energy	14	12	7
Dietary fibre, g per head per day	20	25	30
Salt, g per head per day	12	11	9
Energy	No change		
Protein	No recommendation		
Cholesterol	No recommendation		
Alcohol, % energy	6	5	4

Source: NACNE, 1983

The government of the day was somewhat nonplussed by the report of the NACNE group and immediately distanced itself by labelling the report 'unofficial'.

However, nine months later in July 1984, the official report by COMA (Committee on Medical Aspects of Food Policy) on 'Diet and Cardiovascular Disease' was published. The recommendations were essentially similar to those of NACNE. These were accepted by the government and are effectively part of official government policy. Despite the limitations – the COMA report is restricted to cardiovascular disease and does not attempt to formulate recommendations based on studies dealing with other diseases, such as cancers; neither does it consider positive aspects that would be conducive to good health – both reports have had a significant impact.

The cancer dimension

Although it is believed that diet does play an important role in the development of certain cancers, our current knowledge has not yet reached the stage where definitive recommendations can be made. There are indications that salt may play a role in the development of cancer of the stomach, while a high fat intake may predispose towards cancer of the bowel and cancer of the breast in women. However, it is still not clear whether this effect is due to the fat *per se* or to the high energy intake that usually results from high fat consumption. Furthermore, there is little information on the function of different types of fat in the development of cancers. On the other hand, some research does suggest that fresh fruit and vegetables may be protective as may foods which are high in fibre. Fortunately, all of these are consistent with what is known about the relationships between diet and cardiovascular or cerebrovascular diseases.

In my view, scientists and health professionals must be extremely careful before making recommendations to the public as a whole.

First, they must be reasonably confident that the recommendations do apply to everyone and that there is sound evidence that, if followed, they will be effective. Scientists are especially vulnerable to the criticism that they are always changing their minds.

Second, any recommendations specifically related to cancers must fit in with recommendations based on other research, especially that on cardiovascular diseases. It is quite intolerable to be advising the public to change their diet in one way because of concern about a particular disease and in a completely different way for other reasons.

In recent years, there has been a significant shift in eating patterns as shown by:

- increase in consumption of low-fat milks;

- increase in consumption of low-fat spreads and polyunsaturated margarines;

- increase in consumption of wholemeal breads;

- increase in consumption of high-fibre breakfast cereals

We have now (April 1991) reached the stage where there is likely to be a further push. The British Dietetic Association and the Health Education Authority has just held a major conference entitled 'The Food Network – Achieving a Healthy Diet in the Year 2000' which was attended by representatives from processors, farmers, caterers, consumers, retailers, government, education and the media.

Although there is a measure of disagreement on how to proceed, there is no doubt that all sectors do recognize that healthy eating is an important issue. Even though there are some who disagree with the scientific basis – despite the almost unprecedented consensus of official committees that have evaluated the evidence – there is widespread agreement that the moves towards healthy eating will continue and that much of the push will come from consumers and consumer organizations. Furthermore, there are now signs that government has adopted a much more positive stance than in the past.

The role of government

Almost invariably, governments do have a major influence on the food chain. Legislation dealing with adulteration was introduced in the last century, while controls relating to weights and measures can be traced back to the 13th century. However, the major preoccupation of governments has been the need to ensure that there is an adequate supply of food. Shortages can lead to riots and the downfall of governments.

Traditionally, the major difficulty has been the fact that output can fluctuate because of variations in the weather. From the perspective of farmers and growers, a year in which yields are high can result in a drop in price as the law of supply and demand takes effect. Consequently, the net return to the producers can be so low that they cannot survive economically and therefore decide to get out of food production altogether.

Government measures are therefore introduced to control the markets so that farmers have a reasonable income. In Britain, before entry into the EC, there used to be a system of paying subsidies to producers of certain commodities if the market price fell below an agreed level. This had the advantage of supporting the farmers while consumers benefited from the low prices which occurred when yields were good.

Instead, allowing market prices to fall once the agreed floor price is reached, the producers can sell the commodity to an Intervention Board, which is an EC agency. In theory, this system should allow surplus to be taken out of the market when yields are high so that when there is a shortage, the stores can be released on to the market and the prices do not rise to very high levels. Unfortunately, the floor prices have been set at relatively high levels – because of pressure from the farming lobbies which are still quite powerful in some EC countries. This has encouraged farmers to increase their product year after year so that more and more surplus has been accumulating, giving rise to the mountains of grain, butter, dried skimmed milk powder and beef.

Not surprisingly, the Common Agricultural Policy (CAP) is under pressure to change for the following reasons:

- **Cost**. As the mountain builds up, obviously the cost of purchasing increases. On top of this, the cost of storage for the perishable goods also increases. Obviously this can not go on indefinitely and so various measures are being introduced. For example, milk quotas came in at the beginning of April 1984.

- **Power of the farm lobby**. As new technology is introduced into agriculture, the demand for labour is falling. In Britain today, less than 1% of the workforce is actually employed in agriculture. Although there is a higher proportion in other EC countries, especially in Southern Europe, the numbers are declining with a corresponding decrease in political influence.

- **Growth in the power of consumers**. Modern consumers expect to be provided with what they want and increasingly they are demanding healthy food.

As things stand at present, health concerns do not feature at all in decisions that are made about the farm support measures. Basically, there is so much intertia in the administrative structures that they are apparently incapable of making the necessary changes within a reasonable time scale.

An analysis of recommendations prepared by government bodies and professional societies from all over the world shows that there is now overwhelming consensus on what constitutes a healthy diet. An excellent example is a report prepared for the Canadian government in 1990. The Guidelines for Healthy Eating are:

- Enjoy a variety of foods.

- Emphasize cereal, breads, other grain products, vegetables and fruits.

- Choose low-fat dairy products, lean meats, and foods prepared with little or no fat.

- Achieve and maintain a healthy body weight by enjoying regular physical activity and healthy eating.

- Limit salt, alcohol and caffeine.

(Source: *Towards Healthy Eating: Canadian Guidelines for Healthy Eating and Recommended Strategies for Implementation. The Report of the Communications/Implementation Committee*; Department of Health and Welfare, Canada.)

Many of these changes are in line with the dietary recommendations and it is clear from these results that they are having an impact, although the scope for further change is still very considerable. Various approaches can be taken. Here are some suggestions:

A   There should be a strong measure of agreement on the changes required. These should be expressed as *foods* rather than as nutrients. If this has the full backing of the governments and its agencies, i.e. all are singing the same song, then the messages will have authority and may be taken seriously. During the past 20 years, there have been co-ordinated campaigns in Finland to alter the diet which have been extremely successful, as illustrated by the significant decline in the incidence of heart disease which has been achieved.

In particular, general practitioners need to be well informed about the basic principles of the recommendations because the family doctor is especially influential with his or her patients.

B   Governments can take steps to influence the supply by the way in which the price support mechanisms for farmers are operated. Payment schemes for milk can be adjusted so that there is little or no incentive to produce milk with a high fat content. Similarly, payment schemes for cattle can be structured so that there are incentives to produce beef cattle and sheep with lean carcases.

C   I believe that the most effective way of making the necessary changes are likely to be through retailers and manufacturers. In Belgium, the manufacturers of bread were persuaded to lower the concentration of salt in their product gradually over a period. This meant that consumers had time to adjust their palate and were largely unaware of what was happening.

However, in other cases, it may not be possible to alter the composition of products surreptitiously because there will undoubtedly be some change in taste or texture and there will be a need to develop completely new products. Some companies have already done this. For example, McDonald's in the USA have been reducing the saturated fat content of a range of products, including hamburgers. Similarly, the introduction of low fat spreads and polyunsaturated margarines has been very successful. Because the commercial organizations command such a powerful presence by means of advertising and promotion, they have the potential to advance the cause of healthy eating more effectively than anyone else.

There is also now good evidence to show that the promotion of healthy foods can be highly profitable, although there are certain product ranges, especially those which have a high saturated fat content, that will be threatened. Those companies involved are likely to use diversionary tactics, some which may undermine efforts to promote healthy eating. This can be countered if there is sound education in nutrition in schools and for the general public. Nutrition labelling is also important, but is not mandatory. Even when it is provided, manufacturers are not required to give the breakdown of fat, so consumers may not have the information on the amount of saturated fat in the product.

SEARCHING FOR CONSENSUS:
A CASE STUDY OF RECTAL AND COLONIC CANCERS

Allyson Pollock

Introduction

Clinicians everywhere usually base their practice on empirical judgements rather than on scientific evidence. One reason for this is that in many clinical areas there are debates about the way to treat or prevent illness and there is often no authoritative consensus on scientific evidence and its practical implications.

In this paper, one method of developing consensus, that of the consensus conference, will be described and evaluated. The process and results of a recent consensus conference on colorectal cancers held in the UK will be used to illustrate the issues which can emerge around such a conference.

Background

The consensus development process originated in the United States in 1976 (Baratz, 1989). There, it was fairly narrowly focussed on technology assessment, efficacy and safety (Baratz, 1989; Perry, 1988). By contrast, in Europe (where consensus development has been adopted in countries like Holland, Sweden, Finland, Denmark, Norway and Britain) consensus development has embraced a wider range of issues. Holland, for example, uses consensus conferences of physicians as an extension of medical audit to establish appropriate criteria for quality medical practice (Perry, 1988; Stocking, 1985). Denmark, on the other hand, holds consensus conferences on many issues, often non-medically related (e.g. water pollution) and composed entirely of lay people in order to target members of the public and decision-makers in politics and administration (Perry, 1988; Mullen and Jacoby, 1985).

The aims of consensus development

In the US, where consensus development originated, the National Institutes of Health define consensus as 'collective' opinion which is the majority judgement arrived at by those most concerned with a particular technology or practice. In both Britain and America, the formal written aims of consensus development as it relates to health care and medicine are as follows:

1   To review and assess the scientific basis of a medical technology.

2   To provide information concerning the appropriate use of a technology.

3   To contribute to the dissemination of knowledge concerning the technology.

4   To promote public debate.

5   To enhance the quality of health care by promoting change.

The consensus conference method

Consensus development using a conference as the main tool contains elements of three basic models:

*   the judicial process, in which testimony is heard and evaluated by a jury

*   the scientific meeting

*   the town meeting, where a forum is provided for all interested persons to express their views.

(Mullen and Jacoby, 1985; Jacoby and Rose, 1985)

The main features of the consensus process are as follows:

First, a medical technology or practice upon which consensus, i.e. an authoritative collective opinion, is identified. In the US the criteria of selection are that the technology or practice must (a) have public health and medical importance; (b) be surrounded with controversy which can be clarified by the consensus approach and (c) there must be sufficient evidence to resolve the controversy and it must be amenable to clarification on technical grounds (Guidelines for the Selection and Management of Consensus Development Conference, 1983).

The second stage is to become familiar with the controversies surrounding the topic and to draw together all the relevant literature.

Thirdly, all the groups who have an interest in the topic or technology must be identified. These may be professionals, voluntary groups or lay people. Often, they will have a large investment in the topic under consideration, and their views may be both strong and conflicting.

Next, the important questions which can be usefully deliberated upon at the consensus conference must be identified. These should be identified and then restricted to a manageable number.

At this point, the consensus conference itself can be organized and planned. Suitable experts who can speak at the meeting must be identified and invited. One method is then to choose a multi-disciplinary panel of 12-16 people who are then invited to take part in the conference proceedings as 'jurists'. (These are the people who will formulate the consensus in the form of answers to the questions which the conference is addressing.) Criteria for selecting these panellists might include professional weighting, expertise, the need for consumer representation, the need to include people representing certain agendas and the need to ensure demographic and geographical representation. It is also necessary to ensure

that a wider audience is invited to take part in the conference proceedings as participating members of the 'audience' so that it is a genuinely public event with maximum participation from all parties who might have an interest in the topic under discussion.

Before the actual conference, panellists receive the questions to be resolved together with a literature review and bibliography. They may have a preliminary meeting before the main conference proceedings take place to work out how they should review all the evidence and come to their conclusions.

The conference itself usually takes several days. The first session is usually a plenary session in which expert speakers give evidence to the panellists and to the wider audience which is present. The experts can be questioned by the audience or the panellists. During the second part of the conference, the panellists meet on their own in private to determine their answers to the questions under consideration. They write a preliminary series of statements in response to the original questions in the light of the evidence and opinions that they have heard. This preliminary work is then presented to the wider audience. After listening once again to the views of the audience, a final version is produced. This becomes the consensus statement which is complete and ready for publication and wide dissemination (Guidelines for the Selection and Management of Consensus Development Conference, 1983).

Altogether, the process of organizing a consensus conference may take up to two years. Careful and sensitive preparation and attention to the process as well as to the scientific content is vital if a credible outcome is to be achieved.

Problems with consensus development

The process described may appear uncontroversial and easy to implement. In fact, all sorts of problems and difficulties arise around attaining consensus. There may be controversy about who should take the lead in organizing a consensus conference. The questions which are identified for discussion and resolution may appear to be the wrong ones from the perspective of different organizations or individuals. There may be considerable divergence of interest and perspective amongst those who have a legitimate interest in a topic. Professionals may view some significant elements of a topic very differently from those who represent voluntary groups or those who are service consumers. It may be very difficult to get together a panel which is perceived to be truly representative of all the different interests concerned and so be credible to all those who are taking part. It can also be difficult to assemble a group of experts who are truly knowledgeable and representative.

The panel can easily become dominated by articulate medical interests so that lay and voluntary voices are suppressed or muted. The composition of the panel may be so pluralistic that much of its time is spent in power struggles and consensus cannot be easily gained. A consensus or majority view on any question might in fact finally only represent the view of 51% of the panellists, in which case it will not command respect when it is disseminated. Even when a consensus document is released, it may have little influence on the actual practice of health care and research, i.e. on exactly those areas which it was intended to clarify and influence.

Attaining consensus on colorectal cancers

Many of the difficulties outlined above featured in the British consensus conference on colorectal cancers which was convened in June 1990. Colorectal cancers are the second largest group of fatal cancers in Britain (20,000 people die each year from them). The conference was convened by an independent private body, the King's Fund, at the suggestion of a leading surgeon and organized by a public health doctor.

The first stage of completing a literature review and identifying key questions for resolution was relatively easily and quickly accomplished. There were many powerful, influential interest groups in both the public and charitable sectors who had a strong interest in this area, so it was not difficult to identify professionals who would need to be involved in the conference. However, the King's Fund is committed to gaining consumer involvement in the consensus process and to ensuring that patients and voluntary groups can articulate their needs and, if necessary, challenge professional opinions.

It was very difficult to find consumer advocates who could effectively resist the combined interests of medical professionals and the powerful charities with whom they worked very closely. Many cancer charities have medical professionals at their heads and are basically medically dominated. It was also difficult to find expert speakers on descriptive epidemiology, the natural history of colorectal cancers and economic aspects of this topic. During the conference itself, the consumer representatives were unable to exert sufficient influence for their satisfaction. They felt that they were hampered by a lack of expert knowledge and so had little power to influence the discussions.

Important issues of public health policy and ethics were subordinated to more clinical issues which seemed more significant to the medical panellists who formed half the panel membership. The panel appeared disparate and found it difficult to work together. Panellists were unable to transcend their own interests to adopt a public health approach to colorectal cancers. In the end, the panel made recommendations on issues that it could feel comfortable with and which would allow them to remain in harmony with medical peers and colleagues – thus the opportunity of challenging the profession to new kinds of practice intrinsic to the theory of consensus developments was not strongly developed.

The questions

A public health approach was used to formulate the questions using the structure of primary, secondary and tertiary prevention. The major issues which emerged from the literature, discussion with the planning group and organizations did not necessarily coincide with the professional view, where the perspective tended towards a much narrower focus of interest.

The issues which emerged were:

(a) Neglect of the epidemiology of colorectal cancer. In the descriptive and observational epidemiology literature there are a few case-control studies and even the large European intervention studies currently in progress lack the hard evidence required to support them (Riboili and Sasco, 1986).

   In Britain there is very little research into the epidemiology of colorectal cancer, which may be attributed in part to the alliance of the interest groups and the clinical bias of current research funding. Epidemiology has a low profile. As one leading clinician said, 'It is better to concentrate on screening and treatment issues since there is little likelihood of finding a cause at present.' This may also reflect the clinicians' need to maintain their current high profile in research by demonstrating visible activity.

   The lack of epidemiological input seems to be supported by the clinicians' statistical advisers, who were quoted as being opposed to further case control studies due to the methodological problems.

(b) The second major area of epidemiological concern is the natural history of colorectal cancer which impinges on everyday clinical practice.

It is thought that most cancers of the rectum and the colon arise from polyps. Polyps are small pieces of tissue which form innocent growths inside the bowel. Polyps are very common especially in people aged over 60 years and only a small proportion ever become cancer. For instance, in people aged over 60 years, as many as six out of 10 will have polyps, but only three people in every thousand have cancer. Epidemiologically, it would seem that the risk of cancer developing from polyps is fairly low in people aged over 60 years.

However, the problem is determining which polyps will become cancer. Currently, there are only two real predictors of malignancy. The first is size, i.e. the bigger the polyp, the greater the risk of cancer. The other feature is the histology or internal architecture which can only be observed under a microscope. The group of polyps that are most likely to become malignant are called villous adenomatous polyps. However, these polyps only account for a tenth of all the different kinds of polyps found in the bowel and of these, less than a half will actually become malignant.

There are the additional problems that it may take many years for a polyp to become a cancer and many years for some cancers to cause symptoms and some may not present a lifetime risk. Unfortunately, it is not possible to determine the type of polyp until it has been removed and looked at under the microscope. This means that as many as 25 polyps have to be removed in several individuals to prevent one possible cancer. The removal of polyps carries its own risks as a surgical procedure of bleeding and perforation of the bowel wall.

Currently, clinicians are basing clinical decision-making on the histological rather than the epidemiological evidence for the polyp-cancer sequence. Similarly, the current screening trials which use special strips of paper which can detect blood in the stool (faecal occult blood testing) may yield many innocent polyps. Again the histological evidence is at odds with the epidemiological evidence which demonstrates that only a small proportion of early disease, i.e. polyps, will ever become malignant. However, clinicians are unwilling to take the risk of leaving behind polyps which may become cancer and so possibly many patients have surgery to remove the polyps where it is not necessary.

The natural history forms a crucial area of debate in screening and treatment, as to date, insufficient weight has been given to the existing epidemiological evidence in clinical decision-making.

(c) Molecular research is developing rapidly in two areas: dietary mechanisms for carcinogenesis of colorectal cancer and genetics.

In the field of genetics, the finding of chromosomes linked to familial adenomatous polyposis, a rare inherited form of bowel cancer, has led workers to look for similar links in the common colorectal cancer. There are now suggestions in the literature that a third of all colorectal cancers may be inherited (Dunlop, 1990). This research has already been partly translated into clinical practice with the unofficial expansion in screening through family genetic screening clinics throughout Britain.

The enormous ethical and economic implications of genetic screening programmes for colorectal cancer have not been considered. If the genetic hypothesis is correct, then as many as a third of the total population over 40 years may fulfil potential screening criteria, having a single first degree relative with cancer of the breast, uterus or bowel. This raises major issues about the costs, the benefits and the ethics of *ad hoc* family cancer screening programmes.

(d) Randomized controlled trails are the main focus of funding for clinical research. Statisticians contribute expert advice to the design of clinical trials. Many statisticians believe that the ideal trial design is large and simple, but such trials generally use crude end points such as survival rather than quality of life to determine the benefit of treatments. For most patients with colorectal cancer, the survival advantage conferred by the various treatments is small (weeks or months) and thus the majority of patients have nothing to gain and perhaps a lot to lose from current clinical trials (De Haes and Knippenberg, 1989). At present, quality-of-life measures lag far behind the progress being made in other cancer fields and are not in widespread use in current colorectal cancer trials. There is a positive resistance to the introduction of these measures in the field of colorectal cancer and they are absent from the two major trials launched at the end of 1989 for colorectal cancer by the United Kingdom Central Committee for Cancer Research (UKCCCR).

(e) Patient involvement. The lack of patient involvement at all stages, from the spending of research money to consultation over treatment and screening programmes, emerged as an issue. At all stages of the conference process, it was difficult to find and involve patients.

The major charitable organizations were in the main professionally led, the consumers within those organizations reflecting the professional view. Advertising through the national press and circulating self-help groups with the conference details eventually encouraged a response.

Thus the four questions that eventually evolved were:

1 Would the detection and treatment of polyps reduce the incidence of cancer of the colon and rectum?

2   What preventive measures are there that will safely reduce the incidence and mortality of cancer of the colon and rectum?

3   How effective are current treatments for cancer of the colon and rectum at improving survival and quality of life?

4   What is the direction for future research?

Struggling to reach a consensus

In theory, consensus should include pluralism and public participation. In practice, the colorectal consensus conference described here unwittingly allowed large charitable organizations and medical professionals to dominate the search for consensus. However, after a considerable amount of hard work by the conference organisers and all the panellists and the representatives of relevant interest groups, a consensus statement was hammered out in answer to key questions.

Consensus statement on colorectal cancers

1   **Would the detection and treatment of polyps reduce the incidence of cancer of the colon and rectum?**

   There is no case for colonoscopic screening on a population basis.

   We recommend that the use of colonoscopy in the asymptomatic individual is justified only in those with a high genetic risk of developing cancer and in the follow-up of some of those patients who have had a symptomatic adenoma previously removed endoscopically.

   We recommend that in the symptomatic patient with a polyp the whole of the large bowel is examined and polyps greater than 5mm in diameter are removed.

   Follow-up is not indicated for patients with a single small tubular rectal adenoma and those over the age of 75. Those

individuals with a large adenoma or any type of multiple adenomas should undergo colonoscopic surveillance at 3 to 5 yearly intervals.

We recommend that in order to deal adequately with the existing demands of symptomatic individuals and screening of high-risk groups, provision for colonoscopic services, including training, needs to be improved.

2   **What preventative measures are there which will safely reduce the incidence and mortality of cancer of the colon and rectum?**

   The evidence is not strong enough to recommend dietary changes.

   We recommend that no decision on the introduction of faecal occult blood population screening is made before 1995.

   We recommend that a comprehensive family history is taken as part of the assessment of all individuals with colorectal cancer.

   We recommend that, given the number of people involved and the resource consequences, such screening must be evaluated.

   Faecal occult blood testing is of no value in the assessment of the symptomatic patient in general practice because of its low specificity and sensitivity.

3   **How effective are current treatments for cancer of the colon and rectum at improving survival and quality of life?**

   We recommend that each district should have at least one colorectal surgeon. Proper local referral and treatment protocols should be developed for both elective and emergency colorectal surgery.

   Those patients who do require a temporary or permanent colostomy will continue to need the support of specialist stoma nurses.

   Standards of reporting have recently been outlined by the United Kingdom Central

Committee for Cancer Research (UKCCCR) and should be adhered to.

We recommend that surgeons enter suitable patients into the AXIS national trial.

Follow-up is expensive and studies of its efficacy, organization, frequency and new methods of detection are needed.

These tests have not been used in trials of colorectal cancer therapy, and must be used routinely in the future.

It is critical that measures of outcome are properly audited, and made available to the general public.

Regional cancer registries provide invaluable information and should be supported.

4 **What is the direction for future research?**

(a) Study the natural history of the adenoma, dysplasia and cancer, and the effects of intervention.

(b) Study the molecular biology of colorectal cancer.

(c) Hereditary factors – study the evaluation of the practical and social implications of surveillance of high-risk families.

(d) The development of more sensitive tests of the physical and biological activity of tumours in order to facilitate the accurate pre and post-operative staging of colorectal cancer.

(e) The development of new treatments to improve survival and quality-of-life.

(f) The use of validated quality of life measures in all clinical trials of colorectal cancer therapy.

(g) Studies that will provide insights into the patients' experiences of colorectal cancer, its treatment and the impact on their lives.

Conclusion

Achieving consensus is a difficult and lengthy process which, as yet, has had limited effects on clinical health care and medical practice.

There are real barriers to public and professional co-operation and participation in this process which still have to be satisfactorily resolved. In the United States, medical domination and a narrow emphasis on the assessment of technology using scientific and technical criteria alone means that consensus-seeking can become a rather barren activity. Striving to understand the scientific basis of a technology alone rules out other important issues such as prevention, economics, ethics and consumer representation. In addition, it is not clear whether consensus statements are made to change practice or merely to inform it.

Experience of consensus development in Britain and throughout Europe reveals a more multi-disciplinary approach to consensus development. This may be a strength as it attempts to involve consumers and policy-makers. Potentially, a population-based perspective can emerge from this and unduly narrow professional and specialist viewpoints can be put into proportion. However, this approach also has its weaknesses. The involvement of consumers and non-specialists in consensus development may bring into question the authority of any consensus statement amongst the specialist audiences whose behaviour it is designed to affect. The aims, methods and effects of consensus development are themselves still developing.

References

Baratz, S.R. (1989) *Profile for the consensus development programme in the United States.* International workshop on consensus development for medical technology assessment. King's Fund Centre, London.

De Haes, J.C. and Knippenberg, F.C.E. (1989) Quality of life – instruments for cancer patients: Babel's tower revisited., *J. Clin. Epidemiol.* **42** (12), 1239–1241.

Dunlop, M.G. (1990) Inheritance of colorectal cancer susceptibility., *Br. J. Surg.* **77**, 245.

Guidelines for the Selection and Management of Consensus Development Conferences, (1983) Bethesda, MD, NIH.

Jacoby, I. and Rose, M. (1985) Transfer of information and its impact on medical practice: the US experience, *International Journal of Technology Assessment in Health Care* **1**(2), 420–432.

Mullen, F. and Jacoby, I. (1985) The town meeting for technology: the maturation of consensus conferences, *JAMA* **254**, 1068–1072.

Perry, S. (1988) The NIH consensus development program : a decade later, *New Engl. J. Med.* **317**(8), 485–488.

Riboili, E. and Sasco, A.J. (1986) Current hypothesis on the aetiology of colorectal cancer: critical review of the epidemiological evidence, *Médecine Sociale et Préventive (France)* **31**, 78–80.

Stocking, B. (1985) First consensus development conference in United Kingdom: on coronary artery bypass grafting, *Br. Med. J.* **291**, 713–716.

INDEX